JOHNS HOPKINS

Manual of Gastrointestinal Endoscopic Procedures

Second Edition

JOHNS HOPKINS

Manual of Gastrointestinal Endoscopic Procedures

Second Edition

Jeanette Ogilvie, RN, BSN, CGRN
Lisa M. Hicks, RN, BSN, CGRN
Anthony N. Kalloo, MD

Johns Hopkins University
Department of Gastroenterology
Baltimore, Maryland

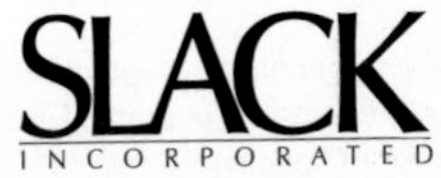

Delivering the best in health care information and education worldwide

6900 Grove Road • Thorofare, NJ 08086

www.slackbooks.com

ISBN: 978-1-55642-810-4

Copyright © 2008 by SLACK Incorporated

All rights reserved. No part of this book may be reproduced, stored in a retrieval system or transmitted in any form or by any means, electronic, mechanical, photocopying, recording or otherwise, without written permission from the publisher, except for brief quotations embodied in critical articles and reviews.

The procedures and practices described in this book should be implemented in a manner consistent with the professional standards set for the circumstances that apply in each specific situation. Every effort has been made to confirm the accuracy of the information presented and to correctly relate generally accepted practices. The authors, editor, and publisher cannot accept responsibility for errors or exclusions or for the outcome of the material presented herein. There is no expressed or implied warranty of this book or information imparted by it. Care has been taken to ensure that drug selection and dosages are in accordance with currently accepted/recommended practice. Due to continuing research, changes in government policy and regulations, and various effects of drug reactions and interactions, it is recommended that the reader carefully review all materials and literature provided for each drug, especially those that are new or not frequently used. Any review or mention of specific companies or products is not intended as an endorsement by the author or publisher.

SLACK Incorporated uses a review process to evaluate submitted material. Prior to publication, educators or clinicians provide important feedback on the content that we publish. We welcome feedback on this work.

Published by: SLACK Incorporated
6900 Grove Road
Thorofare, NJ 08086 USA
Telephone: 856-848-1000
Fax: 856-848-6091
www.slackbooks.com

Contact SLACK Incorporated for more information about other books in this field or about the availability of our books from distributors outside the United States.

Ogilvie, Jeanette, 1949-
Johns Hopkins manual for gastrointestinal endoscopy nursing / Jeanette Ogilvie, Lisa M. Hicks, Anthony N. Kalloo. -- 2nd ed.
p. ; cm.
Includes bibliographical references and index.
ISBN 978-1-55642-810-4
1. Gastroscopy--Handbooks, manuals, etc. 2. Gastrointestinal system--Diseases--Nursing--Handbooks, manuals, etc. I. Hicks, Lisa M. II. Kalloo, Anthony, 1955- III. Title. IV. Title: Manual for gastrointestinal endoscopy nursing.
[DNLM: 1. Endoscopy, Gastrointestinal--nursing--Handbooks. 2. Endoscopy, Gastrointestinal--methods--Handbooks. 3. Gastrointestinal Diseases--nursing--Handbooks. WY 49 O34j 2008]
RC804.G3K35 2008
616.3'307545--dc22

2008010382

For permission to reprint material in another publication, contact SLACK Incorporated. Authorization to photocopy items for internal, personal, or academic use is granted by SLACK Incorporated provided that the appropriate fee is paid directly to Copyright Clearance Center. Prior to photocopying items, please contact the Copyright Clearance Center at 222 Rosewood Drive, Danvers, MA 01923 USA; phone: 978-750-8400; website: www.copyright.com; email: info@copyright.com

Printed in the United States of America.

Last digit is print number: 10 9 8 7 6 5 4 3 2 1

Dedication

This manual is dedicated to the hard-working, devoted physicians, nurses and nursing assistants of the endoscopy units at Johns Hopkins Hospital.

Contents

Acknowledgments

The authors would like to acknowledge the artistic contributions of Michael S. Linkinhoker, MA, CMI, for his medical illustrations and photography. The medical illustrations were reproduced courtesy of the Johns Hopkins Gastroenterology and Hepatology website at: www.hopkins-gi.org.

The authors also wish to acknowledge the following for their contributions to this nursing manual:

Claudia Guilbeau-Brand, RN, BSN
Marcia Canto, MD
John Clark, MD
Regina Crowell, RN, MAS
Cathy Garrett, RN, BSN
Frank Giardiello, MD
Michael Goggins, MD
Linda Hylind, RN, BS
Bronwyn Jones, MD
Sanjay Jagannath, MD
Sergey Kantsevoy, MD
John Kwon, MD
Laura Kress, RN, MAS
Mary Jo Longo, RN, BSN
Laurie McClelland, RN, BSN
Frank Milligan, MD
Gerard Mullin, MD
Christine Smith, RN, MSN
Jean Wang, MD
Lori Wroblewski, RN, BSN
Ronald Wroblewski, RN
Johns Hopkins Drug Information Service
Johns Hopkins Hospital Medical Pharmacy
Johns Hopkins Gastrointestinal Laboratory, Patient Handouts, and Procedure Manual

About the Authors

Jeanette Ogilvie, RN, BSN, CGRN has been a gastroenterology nurse for more than 25 years, 23 of which she has been affiliated with the Johns Hopkins Meyerhoff Digestive Disease Centers. Jeanette has been integrally involved in all phases of patient care in gastroenterology. She was the first nurse at Hopkins to perform flexible sigmoidoscopy and is the lead author of the first nursing publication on the use of botulinum toxin in the gastrointestinal tract. Jeanette has lectured at local and national meetings and has been involved in training physicians and nurses in flexible sigmoidoscopy. For the past 2 years she has served as one of the course directors for the Annual GI nursing Symposium in Las Vegas, Nevada.

Lisa M. Hicks, RN, BSN, CGRN has been a gastroenterology nurse for more than 20 years at the Johns Hopkins Meyerhoff Digestive Disease Centers. Lisa is also involved in all phases of patient care in the endoscopy suite as well as working for the GI website as a web coordinator. In addition she is one of the research coordinators for the Barrett's Methylation Study. She has lectured at both local and national meetings and has been included in publications about Methylation in Barrett's esophagus. For the past 2 years she has served as the lead course director for the Annual GI nursing Symposium in Las Vegas, Nevada.

Anthony N. Kalloo, MD is a professor of medicine at the Johns Hopkins University School of Medicine. He is currently the Chief of Gastroenterology and Hepatology at the Johns Hopkins University School of Medicine. Dr. Kalloo has a national and international reputation as a therapeutic endoscopist and an innovative researcher.

Forewords

It is my privilege to provide leadership to the endoscopy nurses at The Johns Hopkins Hospital. As the new nursing director for the Department of Medicine, I have the good fortune of working with this talented and innovative group of specialty nurses. I am amazed at all they accomplish, and each year they seem to come up with something new and creative to offer their colleagues.

The endoscopy nurses are committed to patient safety and service excellence. They work collaboratively with the entire team of nurses, physicians, and support staff to offer the best care possible. They have recently embarked on a multidisciplinary approach to improve communication across all team members. They are committed to having respectful collegial interactions so much that they have set new standards and offered training and skill enhancement sessions to enrich this culture. I am extremely proud of the work they have accomplished and how they continually grow the profession to new levels.

Their latest work, the newest edition of this book, is another example of their capabilities, and shows how critical it is that nurses have an up to date resource for this kind of specialty care. Endoscopy nurses must bring a wide range of technical skills, nursing knowledge, and pathophysiology to their patient care. In addition, they provide emotional support to the patient and family, and act as their advocate. This dynamic role requires not only highly developed assessment skills, but solid expertise in interpersonal communication, prioritizing, and critical thinking.

This book is a resource that takes endoscopy nurses from preprocedure to postprocedure focusing on all of the elements essential to delivering excellent patient care from procedure preparation to discharge. Information related to sedation, safe handling of equipment, and additional resources are also included. This edition contains the newest procedures and the most up to date techniques. The detailed pictures and illustrations strengthen the text.

This manual is a key resource for new and experienced endoscopy nurses. It functions as a reference for anyone using endoscopy equipment and will contribute to improving the care delivered to patients undergoing these procedures.

Karen K. Davis, RN, MS
Director of Nursing, Department of Medicine
The Johns Hopkins Hospital
Baltimore, Maryland

Forewords

It is my absolute pleasure to write a foreword for the new edition of the *Johns Hopkins Manual of Gastrointestinal Endoscopic Procedures*. I have had the pleasure of working with the consummate professionals in endoscopy over the last decade and a half. Over that period, the demands of endoscopy nursing have become more manifest in holding true to combining a wide variety of elements to provide good care. Gastrointestinal endoscopy nursing is the quintessential example of the complete care process during a patient care cycle combining both the basics inpatient care with the sophistication required to manage conscious sedation and perform endoscopic procedures. The evolution of endoscopy into a more therapeutic endeavor has resulted in a need for a wider diversity of skills necessary to choreograph the patient care process cycle in endoscopy. The demands for more efficiency while maintaining the utmost standards in patient care makes the timing of this edition of the manual even more germane.

The amount of comprehensive information packaged in a palatable easy to read format is simply impressive. The manual achieves a wonderful balance between a reference text and a practical "go to" manual. This manual is a "must have" for those who are newly exposed to the endoscopy unit. It will be a very useful tool for the nurse who is new to the endoscopy unit and veterans alike. Endoscopy nurse managers, physician leaders in endoscopy suites, and administrators will also find this manual useful. It contains all the rudiments necessary for developing skill set guides and standard operating procedures manuals for any units or operating rooms involved in gastrointestinal endoscopy

The authors have combined a number of different stakeholder perspectives to give us this very well written manual. This manual provides us with a tool for fast tracking the acquisition of a comprehensive foundation knowledge base and a tool for consolidating that cognitive knowledge base. The authors deserve hearty congratulations for pulling this together. Readers who are involved with and in the complex but rewarding choreography that is required in gastrointestinal endoscopy will enjoy "dancing" with this manual.

Patrick I. Okolo III, MD, MPH
Chief, Gastrointestinal Endoscopy
Assistant Professor of Medicine
The Johns Hopkins Hospital
Baltimore, Maryland

INTRODUCTION

This manual is intended as a quick reference for users of the gastrointestinal endoscopy unit. It may be helpful for nurses who have the responsibility of preparing patients for endoscopic procedures. It provides endoscopic preparation regimens to facilitate the correct instruction of patients, reducing the likelihood of unsuccessful procedures. This manual should be regarded as a reference; deference should always be given to the patients' physician preferences.

We have provided the definitions and indications for common endoscopic procedures along with listings of necessary equipment. We have used photographs/illustrations in place of detailed descriptions. (Individual employers should provide in-service training on all equipment being utilized by employees in their facility.) Nursing care before, during, and after endoscopic procedures is outlined. Finally, general guidelines for moderate sedation and equipment disinfection and sterilization are discussed, as well as special considerations for patients with specific medical conditions who are undergoing endoscopy.

Chapter 1

The Changing World Of Gastrointestinal Endoscopy

The beginnings of endoscopy are said to have taken place when Adolph Kussmaul placed a rigid tube into the stomach of a professional sword swallower in 1868. Rudolph Schindler, who is called the Father of Endoscopy, published the first textbook of gastroscopy in 1923. The first colonoscopy was performed in 1955 and two years later, fiberoptic endoscopy was introduced. In the third quarter of the 20th century, gastrointestinal endoscopy was considered to be a diagnostic modality. However, the performance of the first polypectomy in 1971 by Doctors Wolff and Shinya probably heralded the field of therapeutic endoscopy. Their findings were ultimately published in a paper in the *New England Journal of Medicine* in 1973.

The timeline of these historic endoscopic milestones illustrates the relatively short history of gastrointestinal endoscopy. It is amazing to think that the first experience of colonoscopy with a videoendoscope was published by Doctors Sivak and Fleischer in 1984. The gastrointestinal endoscopists and gastrointestinal assistants are now faced with a bewildering array of diagnostic and interventional procedures that are rapidly evolving. It is becoming more challenging for endoscopy mangers to handle endoscopic supplies and plan for procedures with the wide portfolio of endoscopic procedures and accessories.

The word endoscopy is derived from the Greek word *endo* which means "within", and *scopein*, which means "to look". Our ability "to look within" and formulate diagnoses have evolved dramatically in the last few years, even since the last edition of this manual. New and exciting diagnostic imaging modalities such as narrow band imaging (NBI) and confocal laser endomicroscopy may become part of standard endoscopic practice.

As a result, new sections have been added to this manual to give you a glimpse of the future with regards to diagnostic modalities. Also included in this new edition is the now widely accepted technique of Bravo pH probe placement which has made significant improvements on patient comfort and tolerance as compared to the previous technique of esophageal pH probe placement. The old techniques of push enteroscopy which are still described in this manual are rapidly being replaced by single and double balloon small bowel enteroscopy. Two decades ago, laparoscopy was a standard procedure performed by gastroenterologists to perform liver biopsy and even peritoneal biopsy. This technique was lost to our surgical colleagues with the advent of laparoscopic surgical interventions. More recently there has been a resurgence of laparoscopy performed by gastroenterologists in the form of minilaparoscopy. The equipment setup and details of minilaparoscopy and liver biopsy have been included in the second edition of the manual.

New therapeutic techniques are also described in this edition. Anti reflux procedures, cryotherapy, and full thickness fundoplication are all newly added therapeutic modalities that have gained widespread acceptance. Endoscopic mucosal resection has been updated with new devices that have been shown to be successful in performing this technique.

As in the first edition, this updated manual will serve to provide you with a quick but comprehensive set-up and how-to technique for most gastrointestinal endoscopy procedures. The future of gastrointestinal endoscopy is bright both from a diagnostic and therapeutic standpoint. We hope that this manual will serve to simplify this rapidly evolving field, and in the process improve the lives of our patients.

Chapter 2

Intravenous Moderate Sedation Guidelines

The delivery of health care in the field of gastroenterology has become more complex and diversified. The days of physician-administered sedation and a nurse and/or technician assisting with little or no patient monitoring are gone. Today, the registered nurse (RN) administers moderate sedation (previously referred to as conscious sedation) assisted by a plethora of monitoring devices. Most gastrointestinal (GI) units staff a physician, RN, and technician in the room. In some instances there are two nurses in attendance.

The Society of Gastrointestinal Nurses and Associates, Inc (SGNA) has outlined a position statement regarding the administration of intravenous moderate sedation to patients undergoing endoscopy. While this position statement provides an appropriate guideline for moderate sedation, it is important for the nurse to follow the guidelines of his or her own state board of nursing and hospital accreditation agency. The SGNA statement maintains that RNs trained and experienced in gastroenterology nursing and endoscopy be given the responsibility of administration and maintenance of sedation and analgesia by order of a physician. The RN is responsible for the administration of reversal agents also prescribed by the physician.

The nurse must be knowledgeable about the pharmacology of drugs used for sedation; their indications, contraindications, mechanism of actions; as well as drugs used to reverse their actions. Additionally, the

RN must have the knowledge and skills needed to assess, diagnose, and intervene in case of complications.

The SGNA recommends that two RNs or one RN and a trained associate be present with the physician in each procedure room to handle the equipment proficiently. During endoscopic procedures, the nurse provides sedation and monitors the patient while an associate assists with the procedure.

American Society of Anesthesiologists Classification

The American Society of Anesthesiologists (ASA) classification is useful in characterizing a patient's ability to tolerate sedation, anesthesia, and stress. Physicians should use this six-step classification to determine if moderate sedation can be accomplished without causing harm to the patient:

- Class I: The patient is healthy and has no underlying organic disease. This is the typical patient seen in an outpatient or free-standing endoscopy center for a diagnostic esophagogastroduodenoscopy (EGD) or colonoscopy.
- Class II: The patient has mild-to-moderate systemic disease that does not interfere with daily routines. Examples: hypertension with a history of coronary artery bypass graft surgery without symptoms; well-controlled asthma, anemia, or diabetes; age older than 70 years; and pregnancy.
- Class III: Severe systemic disturbance such as diseases from any cause, poorly controlled hypertension, poorly controlled diabetes mellitus, symptomatic respiratory disease, such as asthma or chronic obstructive pulmonary disease, and massive obesity.
- Class IV: Life-threatening severe systemic disorders such as unstable angina, debilitating respiratory disease, and end-stage renal disease.
- Class V: Moribund with little chance of survival.
- Class VI: Emergent; any patient who must undergo emergent endoscopy.

Definition of Moderate Sedation

Moderate sedation and analgesia refers to the drug-induced state that allows the patient to tolerate unpleasant sensations while still maintaining control of protective reflexes. The ability to respond purposefully to tactile and verbal stimulation is within the patient's control.

Principles of Moderate Sedation

The following principles of moderate sedation should be followed in all settings when performing endoscopy.

Preprocedure

- Individuals responsible for delivering moderate sedation and patient assessment should be trained in basic cardiac life support.
- It is recommended that a person with advanced cardiac life support training be accessible and on the premises.
- The nurse administering sedation and analgesia should be familiar with all medication actions, dosages, recommendations for titration, side effects, and reversal medications.
- Competency for administration of analgesia and sedation should be a part of orientation for all those who administer moderate sedation. The following is a list of the current criteria:
  1. Demonstrate acquired knowledge of anatomy, physiology, pharmacology, and complications related to intravenous sedation and analgesia.
  2. Demonstrate assessment skills during intravenous sedation, analgesia, and recovery.
  3. Understand the principles of oxygen delivery, respiratory physiology, transport, and uptake.
  4. Demonstrate proficiency in airway management, including the ability to use oxygen-delivery devices.
  5. Have knowledge of potential complications of intravenous sedation and analgesia in relation to the type of medication administered.
  6. Demonstrate skills to assess, diagnose, and intervene in situations consistent with institutional protocols and guidelines.
  7. Be knowledgeable regarding age-specific needs of patient populations under the staff members' care.

Intraprocedure

- Throughout the procedure, verbal reassurance should be provided to the patient. This may improve patient tolerance and decrease the sedation required.

- Continued patient assessment and monitoring of physiologic parameters (eg, vital signs, cardiac rhythm, and oxygen saturation), level of comfort, warmth and dryness of skin, and level of consciousness.
- Vital signs should be documented at baseline and at least every 2 minutes during the initial sedation. After administration of the initial sedation, vital signs should be documented at 15-minute intervals unless the patient's condition warrants more frequent monitoring.
- Reversal medications should be readily available but not routinely administered.

Postprocedure

- Monitoring may be discontinued when the patient's vital signs return to baseline or other criteria established by the individual institution.

Definition of Deep Sedation

Deep sedation and analgesia refers to the drug-induced depression of consciousness during which sedatives or a combination of sedatives and analgesic medications and/or anesthetizing agents are administered. Deep sedation limits the ability of the patients to maintain protective reflexes, ie, airway, breathing, coughing. The ability to respond to verbal and tactile stimuli is compromised.

Principles of Deep Sedation

The following principles of deep sedation should be followed in all settings when performing endoscopy. Since sedation exists along a continuum, deep sedation may be an unplanned outcome of moderate sedation. Planned deep sedation should only be administered by persons trained in the administration of general anesthesia.

Preprocedure

- Same as for moderate sedation.

Intraprocedure

- Same as for moderate sedation.

Postprocedure

- Same as for moderate sedation.

Actions, Dosages, and Side Effects of Commonly Used Intravenous Moderate Sedation Drugs

In general, the drugs used for moderate sedation and analgesia routinely consist of a combination of a narcotic such as fentanyl (a short-acting synthetic narcotic) or meperidine (a longer-acting narcotic) and a tranquilizer such as midazolam or diazepam. Other benzodiazepines may be substituted depending upon the preference of the institution or physician.

In patients who are refractory to sedation, the physician may request administration of other drugs to potentiate the action of the narcotic, such as promethazine hydrochloride which is a phenothiazine, or a butyrophenone such as droperidol.

Fentanyl

Short-acting synthetic narcotic used to produce sedation or analgesia in patients receiving endoscopy. Fentanyl binds with opiate receptors in the central nervous system, altering both emotional and perceptual response to pain.

- ❖ Dosage: 25 to 75 mcg slowly over 2 minutes, may repeat after 3 to 4 minutes up to 3 mcg/kg
- ❖ Onset of action: Immediate
- ❖ Peak action: 1 to 3 minutes
- ❖ Duration of action: 30 to 60 minutes
- ❖ Side effects: Respiratory depression, apnea, arrest, hypotension, changes in heart rate, dizziness, circulatory collapse or arrest, nausea, vomiting, and constipation
- ❖ Antagonist: Naloxone

Meperidine

Longer-acting opioid used to produce sedation or analgesia. Same action on the central nervous system as fentanyl.

- ❖ Dosage: 25 to 50 mg over 1 to 2 minutes, repeat after 2 to 3 minutes as needed
- ❖ Onset of action: 3 to 5 minutes
- ❖ Peak action: 30 to 60 minutes
- ❖ Duration of action: 2 to 4 hours
- ❖ Side effects: Same as for fentanyl

- ❖ Antagonist: Naloxone (Narcan)

Midazolam

Benzodiazepine depresses the central nervous system at limbic and subcortical levels of the brain. Produces sedative effect, skeletal and muscular relaxation, relieves anxiety, and produces retrograde amnesia. Used in intravenous moderate sedation in combination with fentanyl or meperidine.

- ❖ Dosage: 0.03 mg/kg IV over at least 2 minutes. Do not exceed initial dose of 1.5 mg for patients over 60 years of age or 2.5 mg for patients under 60. May repeat 0.5 to 1 mg doses after 2 to 3 minutes. Usually do not exceed 5 mg total, except in cases of extended duration
- ❖ Onset of action: 1 to 5 minutes
- ❖ Peak action: 5 minutes, gradually declining over 30 to 40 minutes
- ❖ Duration of action: Less than 2 hours. If used in combination with protease inhibitors the half life of the drug is doubled.
- ❖ Side effects: Antegrade amnesia, lethargy or excessive drowsiness, respiratory depression, airway obstruction, laryngospasms, lightheadedness, hypotension, tachycardia, and cardiovascular collapse
- ❖ Antagonist: Flumazenil

Diazepam

A benzodiazepine; same action as midazolam.

- ❖ Dosage: Titrate 1 to 5 mg until desired effect achieved; 5 mg endpoint for elderly and debilitated, 10 mg endpoint for healthy adult.
- ❖ Onset of action: 1 to 3 minutes
- ❖ Peak action: 15 to 30 minutes
- ❖ Duration of action: 2 to 4 hours
- ❖ Side effects: Same as midazolam
- ❖ Antagonist: Flumazenil

Droperidol

A butyrophenone; acts primarily in the central nervous system at the subcortical level to cause sedation and decrease the incidence of nausea and vomiting. No analgesic effects.

- ❖ Dosage: Initial dose 1.25 to 2.5 mg over 2 minutes. Repeat doses of 0.625 to 1.25 mg may be given after 5 minutes of initial dose. Maximum dose is 6 to 10 mg

- Onset of action: 3 to 10 minutes, wait at least 5 minutes to assess full effect
- Peak action: 10 to 30 minutes
- Duration of action: 2 to 4 hours
- Side effects: Hypotension, tachycardia, dizziness, drowsiness, dystonic reactions, Parkinsonian signs and symptoms, severe hypotension leading to cardiovascular collapse; alteration of consciousness may last up to 12 hours. Should be used with extreme caution in patients with risk factors for prolonged Q-T syndrome, concomitant use of antiarrhythmics, MAO inhibitors, erythromycin, haloperidol; age > 65 years; or alcohol abuse.

Promethazine

A phenothiazine, promethazine provides clinically useful sedative, antiemetic, and anticholinergic effects. Used in combination with narcotics to promote a sedative effect, it is possible to achieve optimal sedation with doses of 6.25 mg to 12.5 mg. Recommend diluting 25 mg vial in 20 cc normal saline and injecting in the most distal IV port to lessen the burning at the infusion site.

- Dosage: 25 to 50 mg in combination with reduced dosages of narcotics
- Onset of action: 3 to 10 minutes
- Peak action: 30 minutes
- Duration of action: 75 minutes, but effects of the drug may last 2 to 4 hours
- Side effects: Drowsiness, extrapyramidal reactions, tachycardia, bradycardia, venous thrombosis at injection site, hives, and asthma

Naloxone

Narcotic analgesic antagonist used to reverse the effects of opioids during IV moderate sedation.

- Dosage: 0.1 to 0.2 mg every 2 to 3 minutes until the patient responds. Must be administered in incremental doses in order to evaluate patient response. May be delivered via any route if intravenous access is not available. Lower doses should be used in patients taking opioids chronically and in patients being treated for chronic pain
- Onset of action: 1 to 2 minutes
- Peak action: 1 to 2 minutes

- ❖ Duration of action: 30 to 40 minutes
- ❖ Side effects: Reversal of analgesia, nausea, tachycardia, cardiac arrest, and severe hypertension if not administered in small, incremental doses. Abrupt reversal of narcotic depression can result in nausea, vomiting, sweating, tremulousness, seizures, and cardiac arrest. Narcotic abstinence symptoms induced by naloxone start to diminish in 20 to 40 minutes and disappear in 90 minutes. Not effective against barbiturates and sedatives

Flumazenil

Benzodiazepine antagonist; competes for benzodiazepine receptor sites.

- ❖ Dosage: 0.2 mg over 15 seconds, repeat at 1-minute intervals up to 1 mg. May be repeated in 30- to 60-minute intervals to prevent resedation
- ❖ Onset of action: 1 to 2 minutes
- ❖ Peak action: 6 to 10 minutes
- ❖ Duration of action: Frequently shorter than that of benzodiazepines. Related to the plasma levels of the benzodiazepine and the dose of flumazenil
- ❖ Side effects: Seizures, agitation, dizziness, blurred vision, headache, increased sweating, and arrhythmias
- ❖ Monitor for a minimum of 2 hours after administration to watch for resedation. The action of flumazenil is shorter than that of benzodiazepines and does not reverse the amnesic effect of benzodiazepines

Propofol

Propofol belongs to a class of alkylphenols, sedative/hypnotic, used intravenously for the induction and maintenance of monitored anesthesia care (MAC) sedation during diagnostic procedures in adults. Propofol should be administered only by persons trained in the administration of general anesthesia. Persons administering propofol may not be involved in the endoscopic procedure.

- ❖ Dosage: Initial dose: 20 to 40 mg, followed by 10 to 20 mg boluses to maintain level of sedation
- ❖ Onset of action: 30 to 60 seconds
- ❖ Duration of action: 6 to 10 minutes, with a half-life of 1.3 to 4.13 minutes

- Side effects: Pain at injection site, hypotension, bradycardia (possible during infusion) and apnea (possible during induction)

Ondansetron HCL Dihydrate

Selective serotonin receptor antagonist, antiemetic, used for the control of pre- and postprocedure nausea and vomiting.

- Dosage: For the treatment of postoperative nausea and vomiting, a single 4-mg dose by intramuscular or slow intravenous injection (over 2 to 5 minutes) is recommended
- Onset of action: 10 minutes
- Side effects: Headache; constipation; and the sensation of flushing or warmth, pain, redness, and burning at injection site

Dolasetron Mesylate

Selective serotonin receptor antagonist, antiemetic, used for the control of pre- and postprocedure nausea and vomiting.

- Dosage: 12.5 mg IV at onset of nausea and vomiting
- Onset of action: 10 minutes
- Side effects: Malaise, itching, drowsiness, chest pain, and hypotension

Chapter 3

CLEANING AND DISINFECTING ENDOSCOPY EQUIPMENT

Proper cleaning and high-level disinfection of endoscopes and accessories prevent transmission of infection to patients. Standards for infection control regarding reprocessing endoscopes and endoscopic equipment have been developed by collaborative efforts of the American Society for Gastrointestinal Endoscopy (ASGE) and the Society of Gastroenterology Nurses and Associates (SGNA). Immersible flexible endoscopes have become the standard for endoscopy because of their capacity for high-level disinfection.

Proper sterilization/disinfection of endoscopic equipment requires the following components:

1. *Education and training*. Adherence to the principles of infection control is necessary to maintain a safe environment for patients and personnel. The components of an infection control educational program should include:
   a. The use of standard precautions at all times when coming in contact with blood and/or bodily fluids
   b. Knowledge of the Occupational Safety and Health Administration (OSHA) rules on occupational exposure to blood-borne pathogens (OSHA Law 29 CRF part 1910)
   c. Knowledge of reprocessing procedures for endoscopes and accessories
   d. Understanding the mechanisms of disease transmission

   e. Maintaining a safe work environment
   f. Safe handling of high-level disinfectants/sterilants
   g. Knowledge of waste management procedures
2. *Annual updating and training.* Updating and training is recommended to ensure compliance and competency for updated equipment. The number of personnel necessary to clean and disinfect equipment is based upon the number of endoscopes available and the number of procedures performed daily by the unit. Only personnel with the ability to read and understand instructions should be responsible for the task of cleaning and disinfecting endoscopes and equipment. The responsibility of cleaning and disinfecting endoscopic equipment is best confined to a few qualified and appropriately compulsive individuals. The same personnel should be designated for the task of cleaning and disinfection.
3. *Quality assurance.* Quality assurance programs are necessary to evaluate the effectiveness of cleaning and high-level disinfection. All supervisory personnel should be familiar with principles and procedures of high-level disinfection to properly train assistive personnel. Adherence to the policy must be consistent. The disinfection protocol should be periodically revised and updated. The disinfectant/sterilant must be changed regularly with documentation. Periodically, infection control personnel should randomly culture endoscopes. Organisms found in cultured endoscopes should be reported to the nurse-manager for further action.
4. *Procedure room management.* The procedure room must be cleaned with Environmental Protection Agency (EPA) hospital-grade disinfectant after each procedure and at the end of the day. If the unit accommodates patients with known or suspected tuberculosis, the unit should be equipped with high-efficiency particulate air (HEPA) filters.
5. *Cleaning room management.* Endoscopes should be cleaned in an area separate from the procedure rooms. Specifications for the cleaning room include:
   a. Adequate air flow and ventilation (Follow OSHA guidelines for cleaning room air quality, see Appendix 4)
   b. Large work surfaces, including separate "clean" and "dirty" areas
   c. Adequate lighting and water support (at least drinking water quality)

d. Air-drying capability
e. Hand-washing and eye-washing facilities
f. Hospital-specific spill containment protocol

6. *The Food and Drug Administration* recommends a low-suds enzymatic detergent prewash prior to immersion of the endoscope in a high-level disinfectant/sterilant and 70% isopropyl alcohol. All surfaces should be cleaned with a bleach solution or a hospital-grade EPA-approved disinfectant. Disposable equipment should never be reused. All accessories, which are classified according to depth of mucosal penetration, must be disinfected/sterilized according to the manufacturers' guidelines:
   a. Sterilization is required for accessories that break the mucous membrane, contact sterile tissue, or contact the vascular system (eg, biopsy forceps and water bottles. While water bottles do not come in direct contact with the penetrated mucous membrane the water contained in them does, therefore sterile water should be used in the water bottles.).
   b. High-level disinfection is needed for instruments that only contact the mucous membrane (eg, endoscopes).
   c. Low-level disinfection is used for equipment that only contacts the skin (eg, blood pressure cuffs, pulse oximeters).
7. *Cleaning and disinfection*. The following steps should be observed in the cleaning room:
   a. Standard precautions should be observed at all times.
   b. The endoscope should be wiped down with a gauze pad and water in the procedure room to remove blood, mucus, and feces. Clean water should be suctioned through the suction channel and flushed through the water channel until clear.
   c. All removable valves and caps should be detached before leakage testing.
   d. Once in the cleaning room, the endoscope needs to be examined for leakage prior to immersion in the enzymatic cleaner. Attach the endoscope to the leak tester and turn it on before immersion and during the enzymatic cleaning process.
   e. All channels and the outside of the endoscope should be cleaned and manually flushed with an enzymatic detergent (brushing is recommended for the channels); this is the most important step because the disinfectant will cause "debris" to harden in the channels and outside of the endoscope.

f. After the endoscope is enzymatically cleaned, the channels and the exterior should be rinsed with clear water (when using automatic endoscope washers, clear water rinsing is not necessary).

g. The endoscope should be placed in high-level disinfectant (when using an automatic endoscope washer this step is completed automatically, otherwise all the channels of the endoscope should be flushed with high-level disinfectant manually). Follow disinfectant manufacturers' instructions for length of soaking time.

h. The endoscope requires rinsing with clear water (if doing this manually, all channels must be flushed).

i. The exterior and channels of the endoscope must be rinsed with 70% isopropyl alcohol.

j. The drying process is complete after compressed air is flushed through the endoscopic channels.

k. Endoscopes should be hung vertically with valves and protective caps off to ensure fluid drainage.

Chapter 4

Pre-Existing Medical Conditions and Endoscopy

Antibiotic prophylaxis for gastrointestinal endoscopic procedures is described in the table on the next page. One acceptable antibiotic prophylaxis regime consists of intravenous ampicillin 2 g and gentamicin 1.5 mg/kg (up to 80 mg) 30 minutes prior to the endoscopic procedure, followed by amoxicillin 1.5 g orally 6 hours after the procedure. For penicillin-sensitive patients, vancomycin or clindamycin may be substituted.

Patients undergoing percutaneous gastrostomy tube placement should receive cefazolin 1 g 30 minutes prior to the procedure. If, however, these patients are already on an equivalent antibiotic, no other antibiotic medications are necessary.

Diabetes Mellitus

Diabetes mellitus is a metabolic abnormality resulting from insufficient production of insulin by the pancreas, leading to elevated blood glucose levels (hyperglycemia). Blood glucose levels greater than 200 mg/dL, polydipsia, polyuria, fatigue, and weight loss characterize the disease.

Special considerations during endoscopy:

Preprocedure

- Uncomplicated, well-controlled patients should be instructed to take half their normal insulin dose on the day of their procedure. Patients taking oral hypoglycemics should be instructed to omit their morning dose on the day of the procedure.

Antibiotic Prophylaxis for Gastrointestinal Endoscopic Procedures

Medical Condition	*Procedure*	*Prophylaxis*
Prosthetic valve History of endocarditis Systemic pulmonary shunt Synthetic vascular graft	Stricture dilations Varix sclerosing ERCP with obstruction	Yes
	Colonoscopy and EGD with/ without biopsy/polypectomy Variceal ligation	Physician's discretion
Rheumatic valve dysfunction Mitral valve prolapse with insufficiency	Stricture dilation Varix sclerosing ERCP with obstruction	Physician's discretion
Cardiomyopathy Congenital cardiac anomaly	Colonoscopy and EGD with/ without biopsy/polypectomy	No
All other cardiac conditions (status post coronary artery bypass graft surgery, automatic internal defibrillator, pacemaker)	All endoscopic procedures	No

(continued)

(continued)

Medical Condition	*Procedure*	*Prophylaxis*
Obstructed biliary ducts	ERCP	Yes
Pancreatic pseudocysts		
Cirrhosis and ascites	Stricture dilation	Physician's discretion
Immunocompromised patients	Varix sclerosing	
	Biliary obstruction	
	EGD and colonoscopy with/without biopsy/polypectomy	No
Orthoprosthesis	Any procedure	No
All patients	PEG placement	Yes

ERCP = endoscopic retrograde cholangiopancreatography; EGD = esophagogastroduodenoscopy; PEG = percutaneus endoscopic gastrostomy

- Check the patient's blood glucose with a glucometer on arrival to the unit.
- Notify the physician if the blood glucose level is below 60 or above 200 mg/dL.
- The physician may order 50% glucose intravenous (IV) prior to the procedure for levels below 60 mg/dL. Normal saline should be the IV solution of choice for levels above 200 mg/dL.

Intraprocedure

- Changes in vital signs and mental status, including combative behavior, may be a result of changes in the blood sugar level, including hypoglycemia.
- Glucagon, which is used to produce hypotonic bowel, may cause elevations in blood glucose.
- The nurse must be aware of the complications of diabetes. These include myocardial infarction, stroke, kidney failure, poor circulation, hypertension, and heart failure.

Postprocedure

The physician should instruct the patient regarding the resumption of insulin or oral hypoglycemic medications.

Coagulopathy

Coagulopathy is a pathologic condition that affects the ability of the blood to clot.

Special considerations during endoscopy:

Preprocedure

- Verify patient's current prothrombin time (PT), partial thromboplastin time (PTT), platelet level, and international normalized ratio (INR) if biopsy, dilation, or sphincterotomy are contemplated.
- If PT, PTT, platelet level, or INR are not within normal limits, the physician may order fresh frozen plasma (FFP)/platelets.
- Document the patient's baseline vital signs.
- Document the patient's baseline mental status.

Intraprocedure

Have equipment for hemostasis (see Chapter 5, *EGD for Hemostasis in Patients With Upper Gastrointestinal Bleeding*) readily available for control of bleeding.

POSTPROCEDURE

Monitor for signs of bleeding; eg, a significant decrease in blood pressure, increased heart rate, change in mental status, and vomiting blood.

HYPERTENSION

Hypertension is a common, often asymptomatic, disorder associated with a consistently elevated blood pressure exceeding 140/90 mmHg.

Special considerations during endoscopy:

PREPROCEDURE

- ❖ Patients should be advised to take antihypertensive medications as prescribed with a sip of water 2 hours prior to the procedure.
- ❖ Document the patient's baseline blood pressure and notify the physician if the pressure is abnormally elevated (above 200 systolic and 100 diastolic).
- ❖ D5W (dextrose and water) should be the IV solution of choice or D5/.45 NS (dextrose and half normal saline).

INTRAPROCEDURE

Monitor blood pressure and titrate sedation appropriately.

POSTPROCEDURE

Notify the physician if the patient's blood pressure is elevated.

CONGESTIVE HEART FAILURE

Congestive heart failure is a condition of impaired cardiac pumping manifested by pulmonary congestion, systemic venous congestion, and peripheral edema.

Special considerations during endoscopy:

PREPROCEDURE

- ❖ Patients should be instructed to take cardiac medications as prescribed with a sip of water 2 hours prior to the procedure.
- ❖ Monitor and document baseline vital signs, mental status, and peripheral edema.
- ❖ Although electrocardiograms are not required on routine ambulatory cases, they may be ordered selectively based on medical history and physical exam.

INTRAPROCEDURE

- Avoid fluid overload by monitoring intravenous infusions.
- Be alert for changes in the electrocardiogram (EKG).
- Use intravenous solution of choice, D5W or D5/.45 NS.

POSTPROCEDURE

- Monitor and document vital signs, mental status, and peripheral edema.

CARDIAC ARRHYTHMIA

A cardiac arrhythmia is any deviation from the normal cardiac electrical pattern. The heart beat may be too fast or too slow and may be regular or irregular.

Special considerations during endoscopy:

PREPROCEDURE

- The patient should be instructed to take cardiac medications as prescribed with a sip of water 2 hours prior to the procedure.
- Although EKGs are not required on routine ambulatory cases, they may be ordered selectively based on medical history and physical exam.
- If the patient has an automatic internal defibrillator, it should be turned off for the procedure when using electrocautery if working above the diaphragm. If working below the diaphragm, the automatic internal defibrillator (AID) may be left on. However always follow the policies and procedures of your individual institutions.

INTRAPROCEDURE

- Monitor the EKG for any changes from baseline.
- Have emergency equipment readily accessible.

POSTPROCEDURE

- If the patient has EKG changes during the procedure, EKG monitoring should be continued along with monitoring of other vital signs.
- Reinstate the internal defibrillator if appropriate.

Pulmonary Insufficiency

Pulmonary insufficiency is a prolonged or persistent condition of respiratory dysfunction resulting in insufficient oxygenation or carbon dioxide elimination to meet the demands of the body.

Special considerations during endoscopy:

Preprocedure

- ❖ Assess baseline respiratory status.
- ❖ Determine if patient is a "CO_2 retainer."
- ❖ If the patient is wheezing, a metaproterenol nebulizer may be required before the procedure.

Intraprocedure

- ❖ Oxygen delivery should be maintained at 2 L except for in CO_2 retainers, who may require less or no supplemental oxygen.
- ❖ Monitor the patient for coughing, wheezing, dyspnea, and shortness of breath.
- ❖ If the patient is wheezing, a metaproterenol nebulizer may be required before the procedure.
- ❖ Make sure the patient is positioned properly to enhance maximum lung capacity:
    1. Elevate the patient's head and chest slightly (approximately 30 degrees)
    2. Secure proper body alignment so the torso is straight

Postprocedure

- ❖ Monitor respiratory status.
- ❖ If the patient is wheezing, a metaproterenol nebulizer may be required.
- ❖ If required, oxygen may be administered.

Renal Insufficiency

Renal insufficiency is a loss of kidney function and diminishes the ability to excrete wastes, concentrate urine, and conserve electrolytes.

Special considerations during endoscopy:

Preprocedure

- ❖ Dialysis patients should be scheduled for endoscopic procedures just before regular dialysis treatment.

- If the patient has a dialysis shunt or subclavian central line, avoid using that arm for blood pressure, intravenous fluids, or administration of medications.

Intraprocedure

- Monitor intravenous fluids carefully to prevent fluid overload.
- Monitor the amount of sedation the patient is receiving since he or she may have difficulty excreting the medication.

Postprocedure

- Monitor urine output (have the patient void before discharge from the unit).
- Be aware of the complications of renal insufficiency; eg, hypertension, poor circulation, diabetes mellitus, or a change in mental status.

Chapter 5

Diagnostic and Therapeutic Endoscopic Procedures

EGD

Diagnostic Esophagogastroduodenoscopy

Esophagogastroduodenoscopy (EGD) refers to the endoscopic examination of the esophagus, stomach, and the first and second portions of the small intestine for the purpose of diagnosis and treatment of disorders of the upper gastrointestinal tract.

Equipment (Figure 5-1)

1. Upper endoscope
2. Light source
3. Sterile water bottle and sterile water
4. Biopsy forceps (Figure 5-2)
5. Bite block (Figure 5-3)
6. Topical anesthetic
7. Suction equipment (Figure 5-4)

Additional Equipment That May be Needed

1. Bottles of formalin for biopsy specimens
2. Labels with patient's name and pathology requisitions
3. Cytology brushes (Figure 5-5)
4. Viral and fungal culture tubes
5. Mucus trap (Figure 5-6)

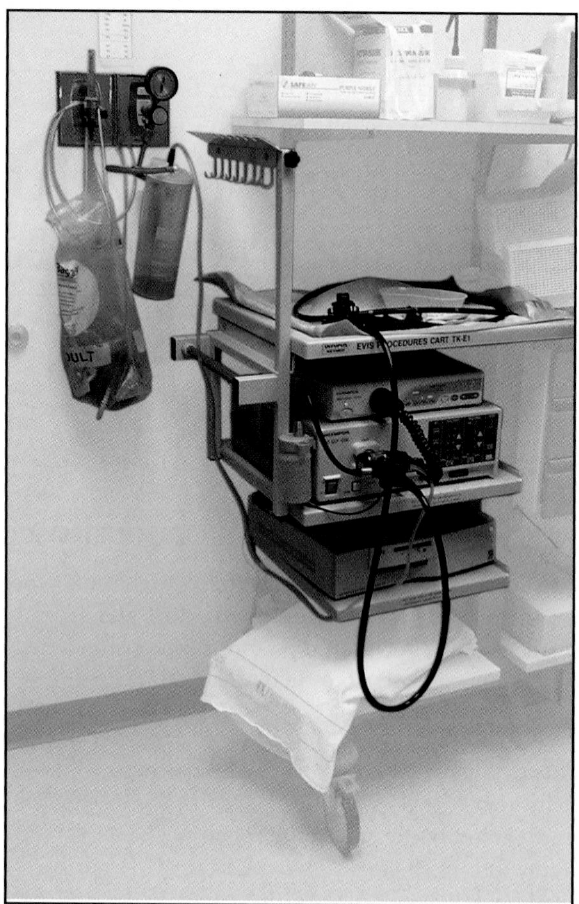

Figure 5-1. Endoscopy set-up.

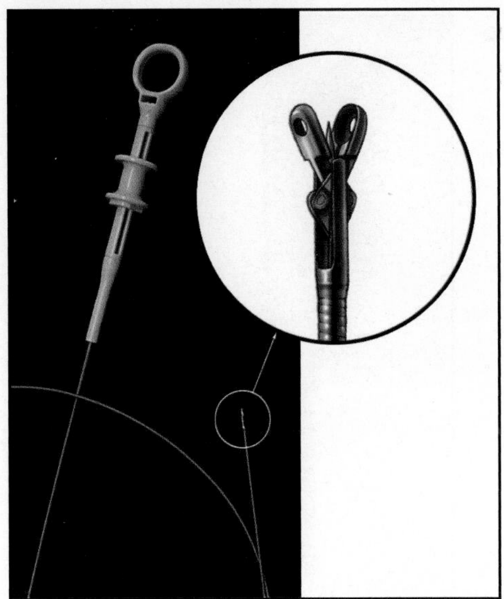

Figure 5-2. Biopsy forceps.

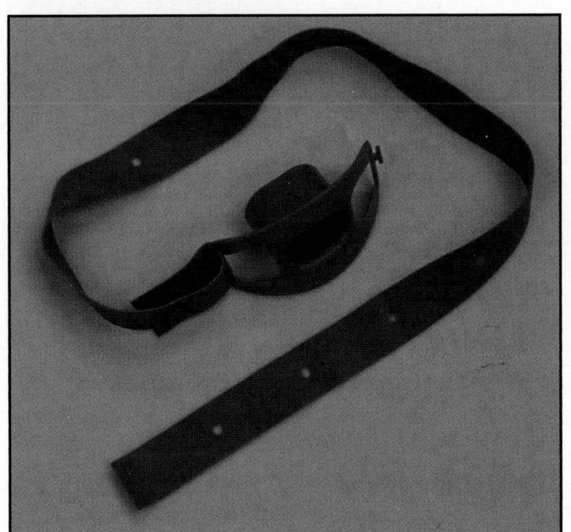

Figure 5-3. Bite block.

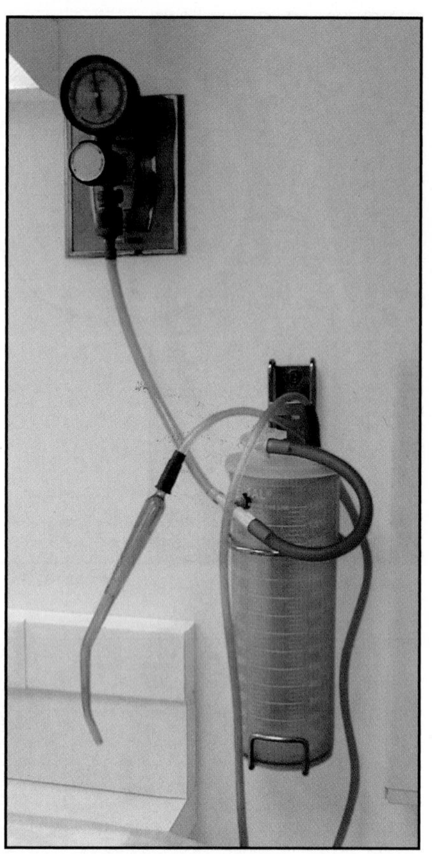

Figure 5-4. Suction apparatus.

Nursing Implications

Preprocedure

- ❖ The patient should have nothing by mouth for 8 hours prior to the procedure.
- ❖ Document baseline blood pressure, pulse, respirations, oxygen saturation, level of consciousness, and pain level.
- ❖ Document drug allergies and daily medications, including dose and frequency.

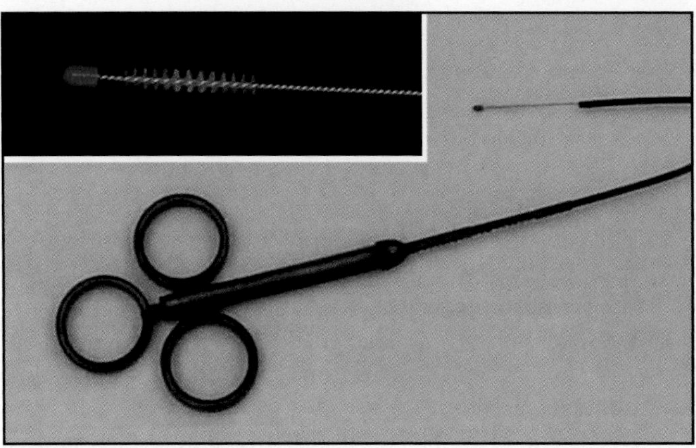

Figure 5-5. Cytology brush.

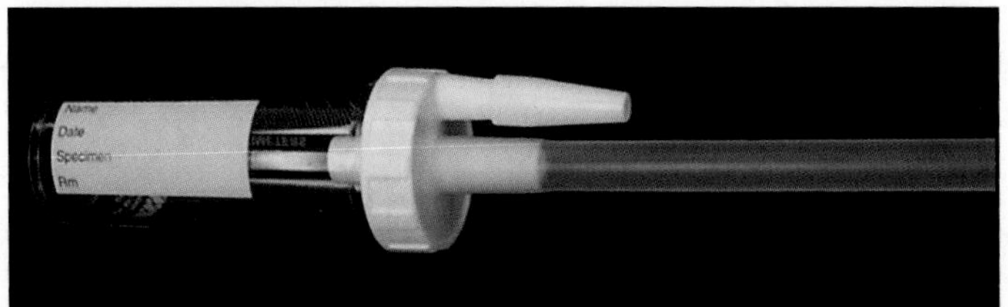

Figure 5-6. Mucus trap.

- ❖ Discontinue aspirin and nonsteroidal anti-inflammatory drugs (NSAIDs) for 1 week prior to the procedure.
- ❖ Start intravenous (IV) of D5/.45 NS (normal saline) or .9 normal saline.
- ❖ The physician should obtain an informed consent from the patient or responsible adult.
- ❖ Obtain medical history from the patient or responsible adult and confirm the completion of a physical exam by the physician.
- ❖ Review the discharge instructions with the patient or responsible adult before sedation is administered.
- ❖ Ensure that a responsible adult is available to accompany the patient home.

Intraprocedure

- Patient positioning (Figure 5-7):
  1. Use left lateral position to facilitate drainage of pharyngeal secretions.
  2. Knees should be bent toward the chest for comfort and stabilization of the patient.
  3. The patient's head may be flexed in a forward position to ease the introduction of the endoscope.
- Patient monitoring:
  1. Document electrocardiogram (EKG), blood pressure, respiratory rate, and pulse oximetry every 2 minutes during administration of sedation.
  2. Document EKG, blood pressure, respiratory rate, and pulse oximetry every 15 minutes during the procedure or more often if the patient's condition warrants.
  3. Pain level must be monitored during the procedure.
  4. Emergency equipment including suction, oxygen, and crash cart must be readily available.
- Topical anesthetic:
  1. Viscous lidocaine swish and swallow or 4% lidocaine spray may be used.
- Additional comfort measures:
  1. Place a pillow behind the patient's back for extra support while on his or her side.
  2. Soothing, calming words of encouragement along with light back massage may improve the patient's comfort.

Postprocedure

- Keep the patient on the left side until fully awake and able to control secretions.
- Monitor vital signs, blood pressure, pulse, oxygen saturation, level of consciousness, and pain level until they have returned to baseline.
- The patient may be discharged home, accompanied by an adult with discharge instructions (see Appendix 3).
- The physician should be notified if the patient experiences vomiting, abdominal pain, distension, or fever.

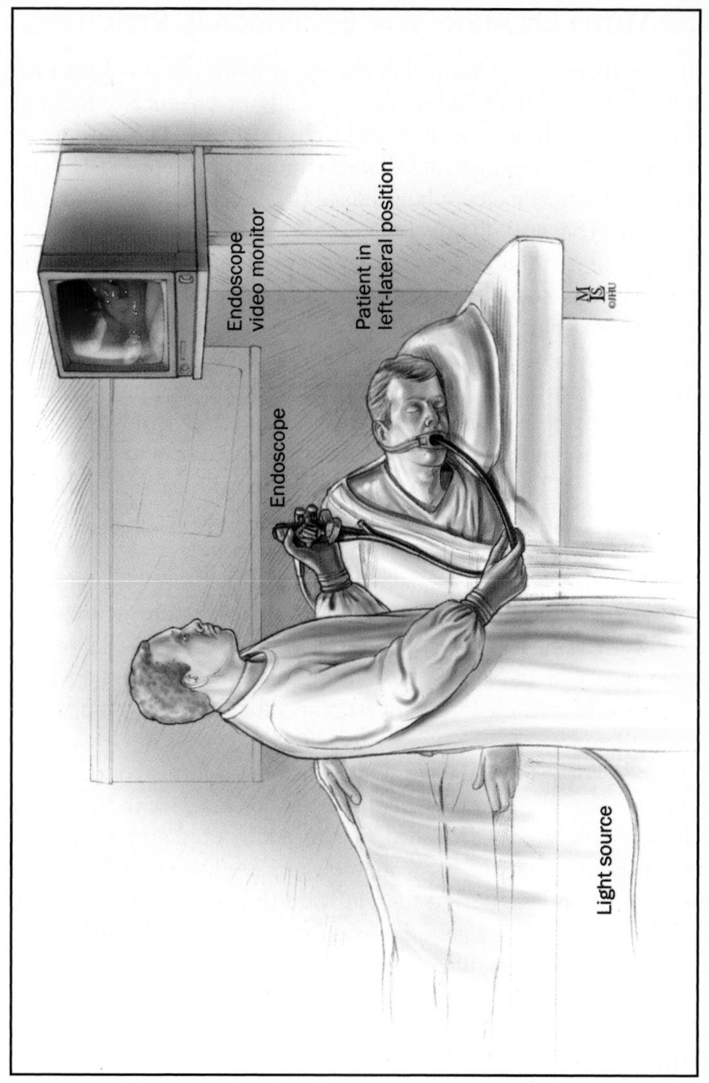

Figure 5-7. Patient positioning for EGD.

Chapter 5

EGD With Dilation for Esophageal Strictures

Dilation therapy is performed in the upper gastrointestinal tract for the following conditions: achalasia, surgically or chemically induced esophageal and pyloric strictures, and webs or rings. The instruments used to dilate strictures include balloons (through-the-scope [TTS] and over-the-guidewire), mercury bougienage (Maloney) dilators, and hollow polyvinyl (Savary) dilators (Figure 5-8).

The type of instrument used is dependent upon the severity of the stricture. Mild to moderately tight strictures can be dilated with a TTS balloon. Fluoroscopy is seldom required, and the risk of perforation is low in cases of benign strictures. Maloney dilators may also be used for this type of stricture. The physician proceeds by beginning with a dilator that can be passed through the stricture with mild resistance and continues to increase the dilator size up to three sizes in succession ("rule of threes"). The physician may continue to increase the dilator size provided that the resistance is mild to moderate.

Achalasia and Savary dilators, both over-the-guidewire, are typically used with fluoroscopy. The achalasia dilator is used only for patients with achalasia (a motility disorder of the esophagus resulting in failure of the lower esophageal sphincter to relax). The balloon dilators are available in a variety of sizes: 30 mm, 35 mm, 40 mm, and 45 mm. The Savary dilator is used for tight strictures that prohibit passage of a Maloney dilator.

The endoscope is initially passed to assess the tightness of the stricture. When using the Maloney dilator, the endoscope is withdrawn and the dilator blindly passed, guided by the endoscopist's finger placed into the patient's pharynx. TTS dilators are passed through the biopsy channel of the endoscope and then inflated (Figure 5-9). Both Savary and achalasia dilators are passed over a guidewire after the endoscope is withdrawn. Achalasia dilators demonstrate a "waist" on fluoroscopy that disappears upon inflation of the balloon (Figure 5-10). The radiopaque-marked Savary dilators can be followed through the stricture with the use of fluoroscopy.

Equipment

1. Same as for a diagnostic EGD.
2. A pediatric endoscope may be used depending upon the tightness of the stricture.

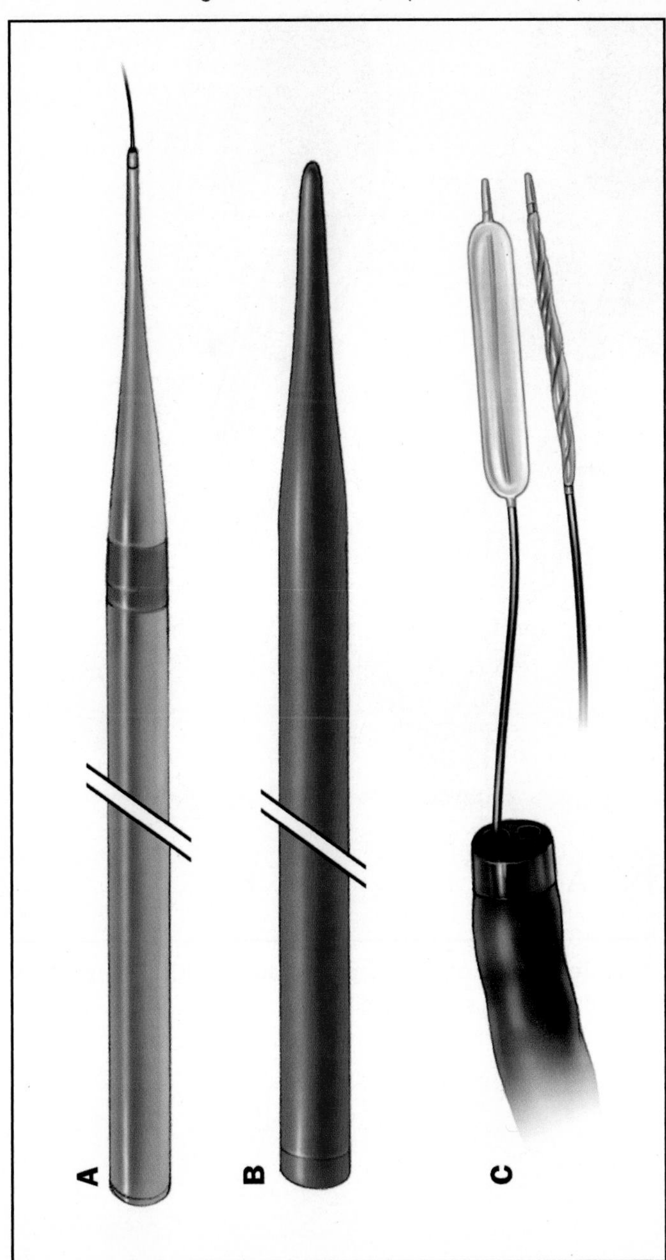

Figure 5-8. Dilators used for esophageal dilation: (A) Savary dilator; (B) Maloney dilator; (C) "through-the-scope" dilator.

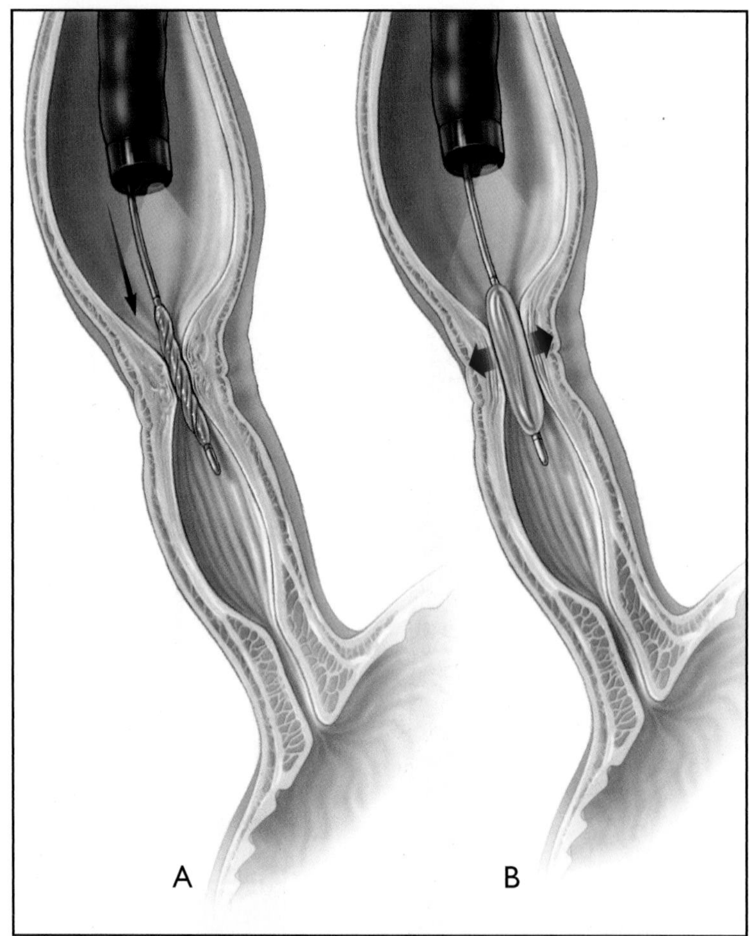

Figure 5-9. Technique of esophageal dilation with TTS dilators before (A) and after (B) stricture dilation.

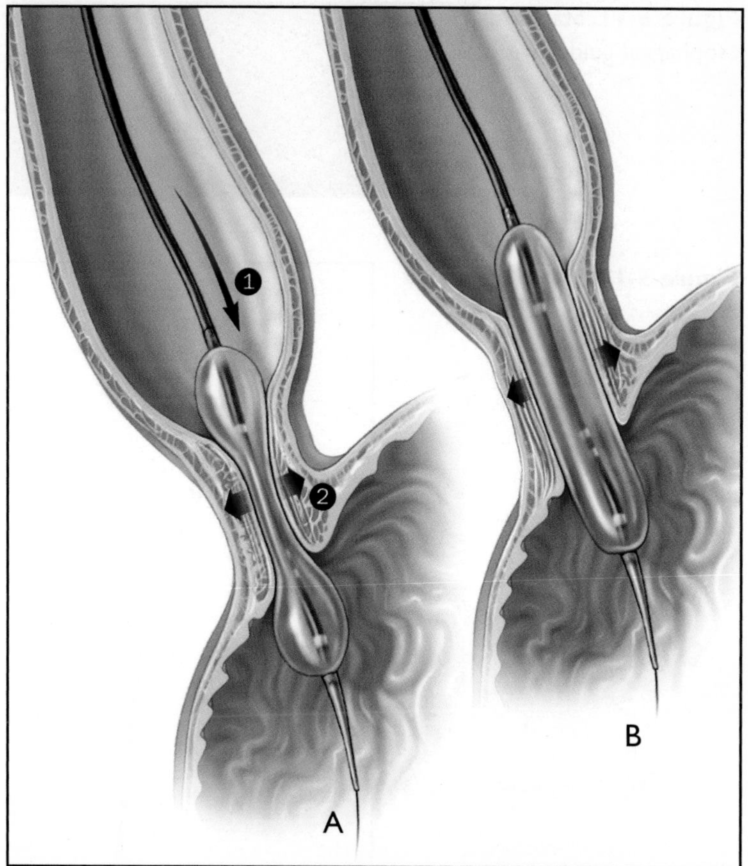

Figure 5-10. Technique of pneumatic dilation before (A) and after (B) dilation.

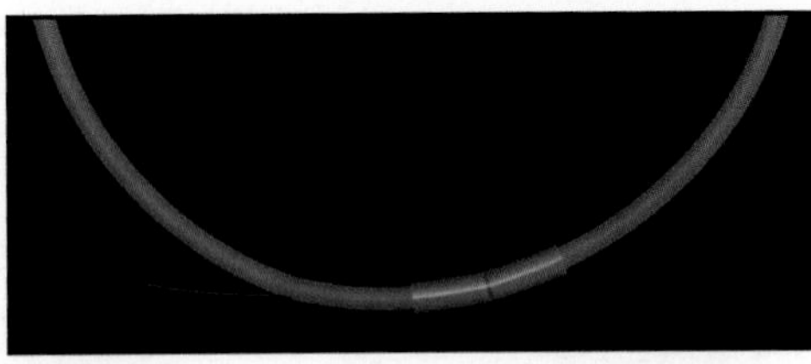

Figure 5-11. Standard esophageal guidewire.

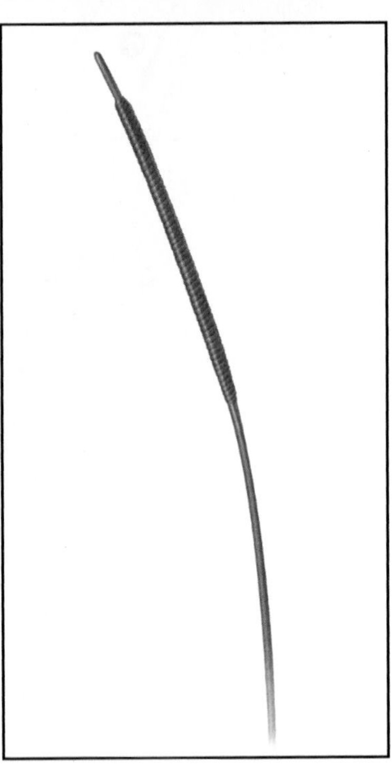

Figure 5-12. Savary guidewire.

3. A large-bore mouth piece may be needed to accommodate a 20-mm dilator.
4. Savary dilators and guidewire (Savary guidewire or any .038-inch diameter guidewire per physician's preference) (Figures 5-11 and 5-12).
5. Fluoroscopy
6. Water-soluble lubricant

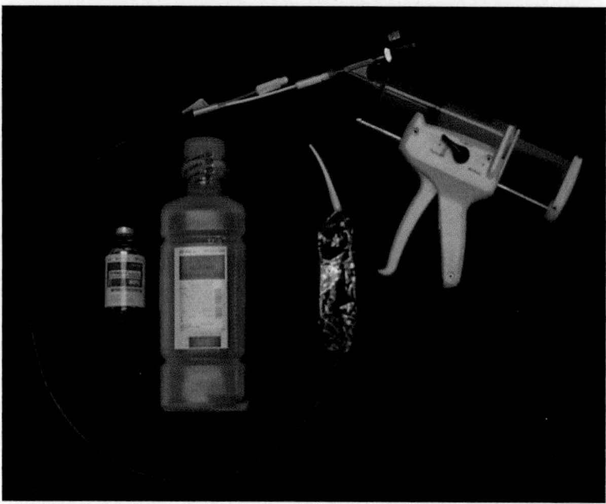

Figure 5-13. Pneumatic dilator gun attached to balloon with agents for balloon sufflation.

Equipment for TTS Dilation

1. Same as for a diagnostic EGD.
2. A pediatric endoscope may be used depending upon the tightness of the stricture.
3. TTS balloons (10 to 20 mm)
4. Dilating gun and adapter with pressure gauge and syringe (Figure 5-13)
5. Water for insufflation of balloon
6. Lubricant (vegetable spray works well with this type of dilator)

Equipment for Maloney Dilation

1. Same as for a diagnostic EGD.
2. A pediatric endoscope may be used depending upon the tightness of the stricture.
3. Maloney dilators (36 to 60 mm, increasing in 4 mm increments)
4. Water or water-soluble lubricant

Equipment for Achalasia Dilation

1. Same as for a diagnostic EGD.
2. A pediatric endoscope may be used depending upon the tightness of the stricture.
3. Fluoroscopy
4. Radiopaque .038-inch diameter guidewire
5. Over-the-guidewire achalasia balloon dilators (30 mm, 35 mm, 40 mm, and 45 mm)
6. Radiopaque half-strength contrast (50 cc distilled water plus 50 cc ionic contrast)
7. Water and water-soluble lubricant for lubrication of dilator

Nursing Implications

Preprocedure

- ❖ Same as for a diagnostic EGD.
- ❖ Anticoagulant therapy may be adjusted or discontinued on the advice of the physician.
- ❖ Prophylactic antibiotics (if indicated).
- ❖ Patients undergoing achalasia dilation should have clear liquids for 24 to 36 hours prior to the procedure since retained food may be present in the esophagus even after a 12-hour fast.

Intraprocedure

- ❖ Same as for a diagnostic EGD.
- ❖ The patient should be positioned on the fluoroscopy table for Savary or achalasia dilations. Fluoroscopy may be necessary for guidewire placement.
- ❖ Savary dilation: The physician may require assistance with the guidewire. The nurse should keep the end of the guidewire coiled and taut while the dilator is passed. The guidewire should not be allowed to slide forward or backward during insertion or removal by paying attention to the guidewire markings.
- ❖ TTS dilation: The nurse will be asked to inflate the balloon to the appropriate pressure. Inflation duration is dependent on the discretion of the physician.
- ❖ Maloney dilation: The nurse should support the distal end of the dilator during insertion by the physician.

- Achalasia dilation: Patient comfort and compliance are aided by bolus sedation immediately before balloon inflation (because of increased pain during dilation).
- Patient monitoring: Same as for a diagnostic EGD.
- Topical anesthetic: Same as for a diagnostic EGD.
- Additional comfort measures: Same as for a diagnostic EGD.
- Some bleeding and increased pharyngeal fluid may be expected during dilation. Frequent suctioning is imperative to prevent aspiration.

Postprocedure

- Same as for a diagnostic EGD.
- Patients should be monitored for symptoms and signs of perforation (chest pain, difficulty breathing or swallowing, or presence of subcutaneous air) following dilation. The risk of perforation is higher in achalasia dilation.
- The patient should be able to take fluid by mouth without difficulty or pain prior to discharge.
- Radiologic studies may be required after dilation if the patient exhibits symptoms or signs of perforation.

Chapter 5

ANTI-REFLUX PROCEDURES

One in 10 Americans suffer daily from gastroesophageal reflux disease (GERD). GERD is a chronic condition that results from an increase in reflux of gastric contents into the esophagus. There are four major symptoms of GERD: heartburn, regurgitation of gastric acid or sour contents into the mouth, difficulty or painful swallowing, and chest pain. Left untreated, GERD can lead to Barrett's esophagus which can lead to cancer. There are three procedures that are FDA approved that can be used to limit the reflux of the acid: full-thickness fundoplication, endoluminal gastroplication, and thermal ablation.

FULL-THICKNESS FUNDOPLICATION

This procedure is used in the treatment of mild to moderate GERD. This procedure allows for restructuring of the cardia and reshaping of the lower esophageal sphincter (LES) by delivering a full thickness suture to the gastric serosa. It is considered a safe alternative to the traditional approach. Two physicians are necessary to perform this procedure.

Contraindications to this procedure and endoluminal gastric plication are: benign or malignant tissue changes preventing secure fixation, esophageal varices, motility disorders of the esophagus, prior gastric or esophageal surgery, persistent dysphagia, unresponsive to proton pump inhibitors (PPIs), and coagulopathies.

EQUIPMENT

1. Same as for diagnostic EGD. Use a 5.9- to 6-mm upper endoscope.
2. Plicator scope: no processor needed (from plicator manufacturer) (Figure 5-14)
3. Savary guidewire
4. Plicator tissue retractor (from plicator manufacturer)
5. Plicator implant cartridge (from plicator manufacturer)
6. Vegetable spray

NURSING IMPLICATIONS

Preprocedure

- ❖ Same as for diagnostic EGD.
- ❖ Document patient coagulopathies on patient chart (INR, PT, PTT).

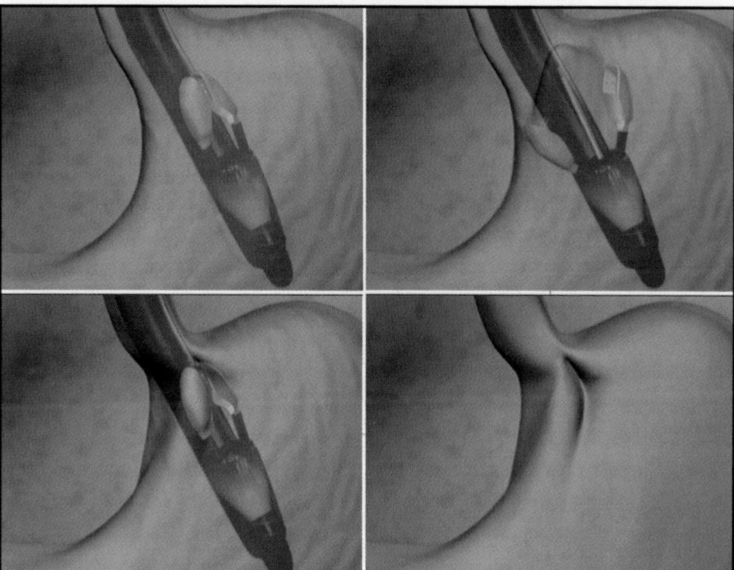

Figure 5-14. Full thickness fundoplicator.

- ❖ Antibiotic prophylaxis as needed.
- ❖ Moderate sedation or monitored anesthesia care (preferred especially if the physician is a novice at this procedure).

Intraprocedure

- ❖ Same as for diagnostic EGD.
- ❖ Lubricate the inside of the plicator scope with the vegetable spray.
- ❖ Check articulation of plicator scope for sufficient retroflexion.
- ❖ Place the clips on the end of the plicator scope as per manufacturer's instructions.

Postprocedure

- ❖ Same as for diagnostic EGD.
- ❖ Patient may require pain medication.
- ❖ Patient should follow a soft diet for 5 days postprocedure.
- ❖ Patient should continue anti-reflux therapy 7 days postprocedure.

Chapter 5

ENDOLUMINAL GASTRIC PLICATION

EQUIPMENT (FIGURE 5-15)

1. Same as for diagnostic EGD
2. Suturing kit (Follow manufacturer's instructions)
3. Guidewire, overtube, and Savary dilator (45 French) or 44 F Maloney dilator
4. Second suction set-up with vacuum pressure of at least 381 mmHg should be consistently maintained.
5. Vegetable spray

NURSING IMPLICATIONS

Preprocedure

- ❖ Same as for diagnostic EGD full-thickness fundoplication.

Intraprocedure

- ❖ Same as for diagnostic EGD.
- ❖ Verify compatibility of endoscopic instruments and accessories from different manufacturers.
- ❖ Inspect endoscopic suturing handle for defects or foreign matter; actuate handle to insure proper working condition.
- ❖ Follow manufacturer's instructions for rest of set-up.
- ❖ Tilt patient's chin upward to facilitate passage of overtube.
- ❖ May need a motility inhibitor during procedure (ie, glucagon).
- ❖ Lubricate endoscope and overtube well with vegetable spray to minimize friction.
- ❖ When removing endoscope from the body, the nurse should keep gentle traction on the suture.
- ❖ Place light tension on the free end of the suture to take up slack as the endoscope is advanced to place the second stitch.

Postprocedure

- ❖ Same as for diagnostic EGD.
- ❖ Patient may need antiemetic postprocedure to reduce risk of disrupting sutures from vomiting.
- ❖ Sore throat may be more apparent from overtube trauma.
- ❖ Abdominal pain may be more apparent from over insufflations during the procedure.

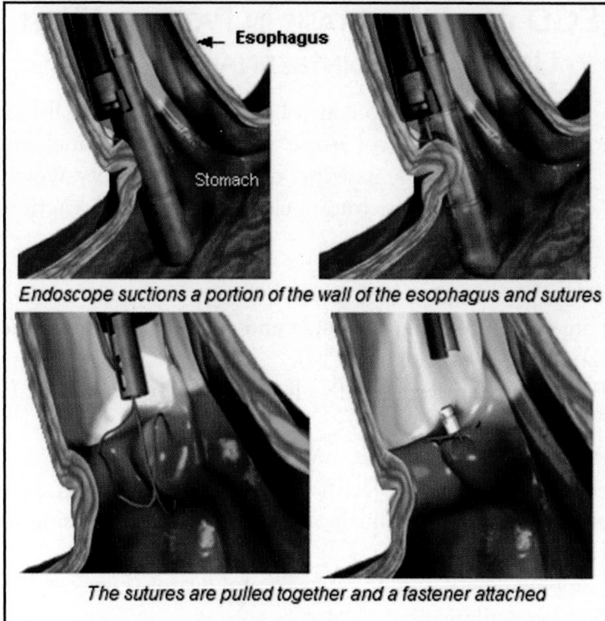

Figure 5-15. Endoluminal gastric plicator.

Chapter 5

EGD for Hemostasis in Patients With Upper Gastrointestinal Bleeding

EGD may be performed to control upper gastrointestinal bleeding. The most common causes of acute upper gastrointestinal bleeding include esophageal varices, gastritis, duodenitis, Mallory-Weiss tears, gastric and duodenal ulcers, watermelon stomach, and arteriovenous malformations (AVMs).

Equipment

1. Large or double-channel upper endoscope (to facilitate the aspiration of blood) (Figure 5-16)
2. Bipolar cautery probe with electrosurgical cautery unit (Figure 5-17)
3. Argon plasma coagulator (APC) (Figure 5-18)
4. Sclerotherapy needle with injectable agents (such as saline, epinephrine, or sodium morrhuate or other sclerosing agents) (Figure 5-19)
5. Clipping device and/or variceal band ligator (Figure 5-20)
6. Suction equipment

Nursing Implications

Preprocedure

- ❖ Same as for a diagnostic EGD.
- ❖ Gastric lavage may be ordered to clear the stomach of blood and food in emergent situations.

Intraprocedure

- ❖ Same as for a diagnostic EGD.
- ❖ Patient positioning: Same as for a diagnostic EGD.
- ❖ Patient monitoring: Same as for a diagnostic EGD.
- ❖ Topical anesthetic: Same as for a diagnostic EGD.
- ❖ Additional comfort measures: Same as for a diagnostic EGD.

Postprocedure

- ❖ Same as for a diagnostic EGD.

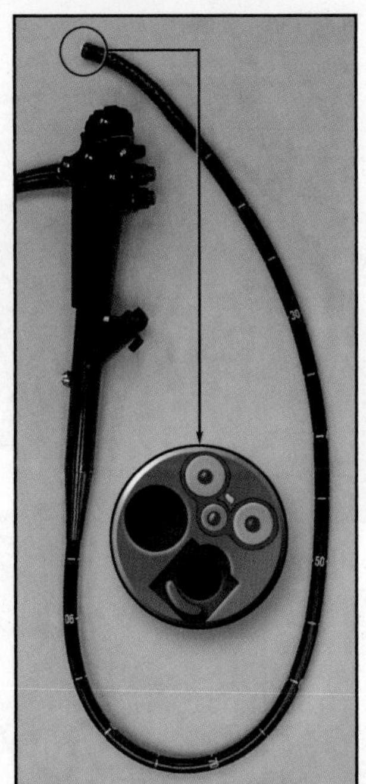

Figure 5-16. Double channel (therapeutic endoscope).

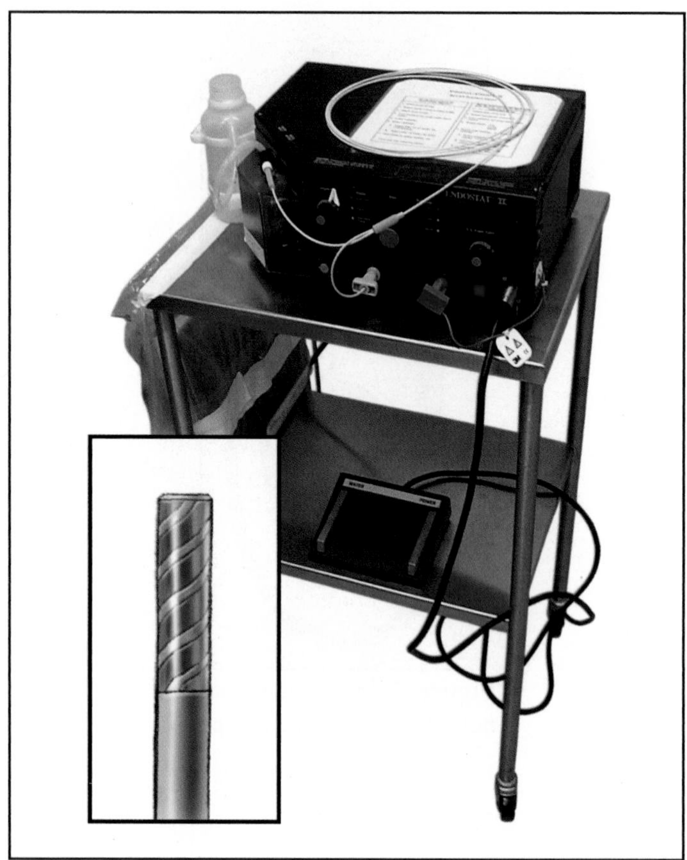

Figure 5-17. Electrosurgical unit with cautery probe.

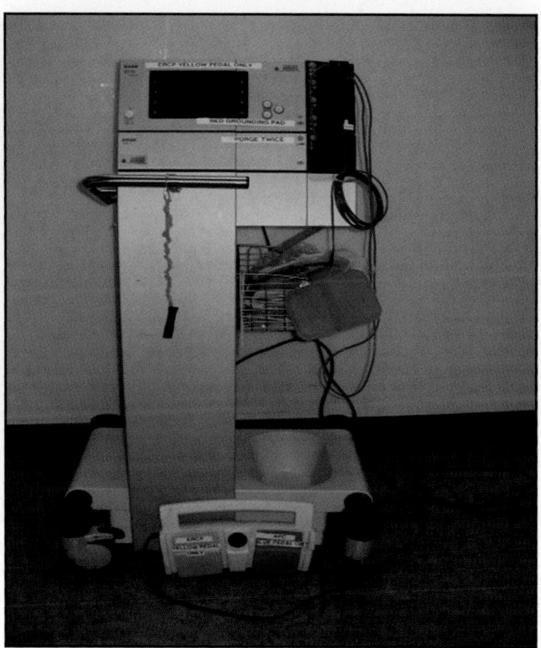

Figure 5-18. Argon plasma coagulator (APC).

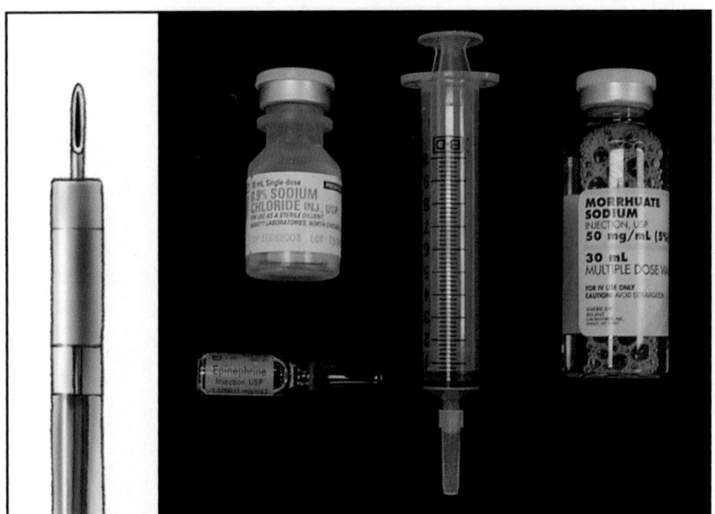

Figure 5-19. Sclerotherapy needle with agents used for injection.

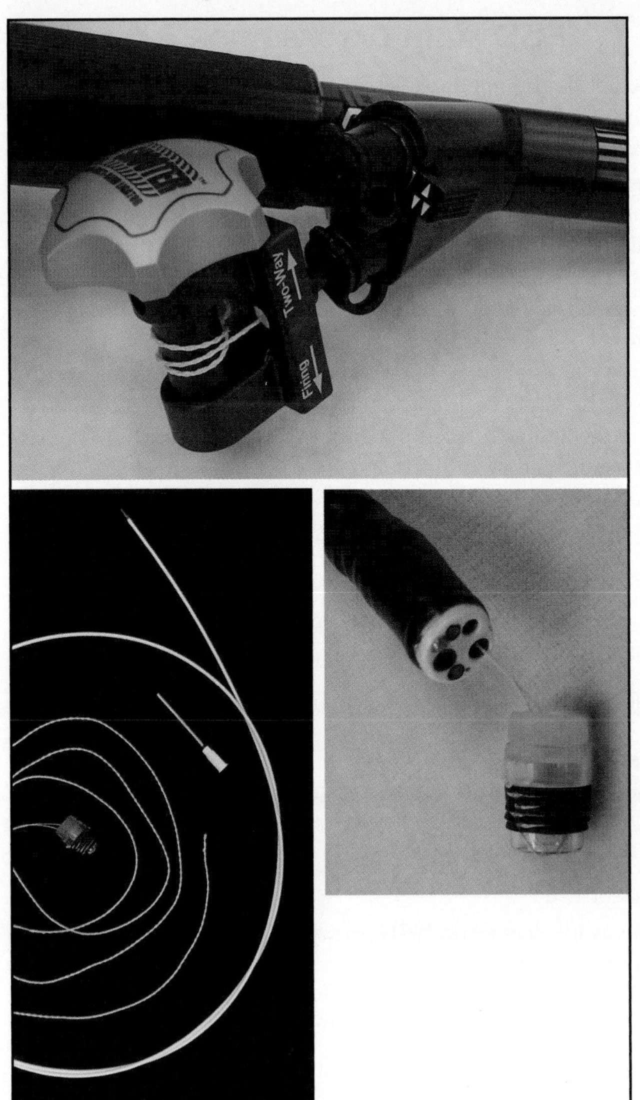

Figure 5-20. Typical band ligation equipment and set-up.

Chapter 5

EGD WITH CRYOABLATION

Cryotherapy is the application of extreme cold to the GI mucosa with either a high pressure device using nitrous oxide gas or a low pressure device using liquid nitrogen at ambient pressure. Cryoablation is performed to remove the dysplastic tissue of Barrett's Esophagus, provide hemostasis of GI bleeding (ie, watermelon stomach), and palliation of gastric neoplasms.

The gas or liquid is delivered through a specially designed 7F stainless steel catheter covered by a Teflon sheath that is passed through the biopsy channel of a standard endoscope. The catheter can deliver pressure of 450 to 750 psi. Freezing is accomplished by the rapid release and expansion of the gas. The lesion of cryotherapy is easily recognized as a white, sharply defined, frozen patch of tissue. After thawing, the tissue becomes engorged with blood and after 24 hours the mucosal layer blisters and sheds. More than one session may be necessary depending on the size of the area being treated.

EQUIPMENT (FIGURE 5-21)

1. Same as for diagnostic EGD, except for the cryo unit and stainless steel catheter.

NURSING IMPLICATIONS

Preprocedure

- ❖ Same as for diagnostic EGD, except for preparation of cryo unit and stainless steel catheter which should be set up according to the manufacturers' instructions.

Intraprocedure

- ❖ Same as for diagnostic EGD, except that the nurse should palpate the abdomen frequently for excessive distention and inform the physician so he can suction the excess gas. Excess gas in the stomach may compromise the patient's respiratory status.

Postprocedure

- ❖ Same as for diagnostic EGD.
- ❖ If necessary make appointment for subsequent therapy.

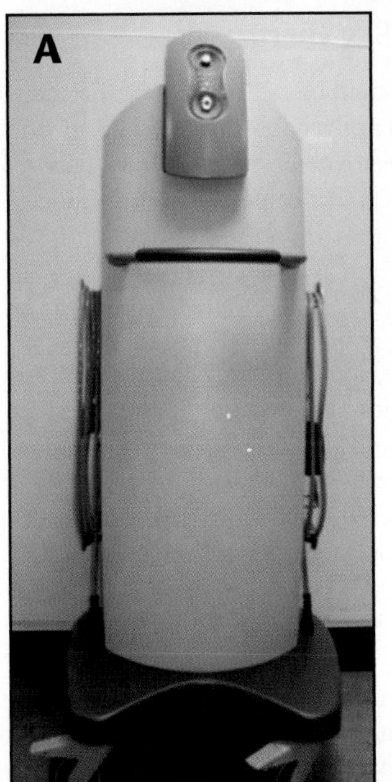

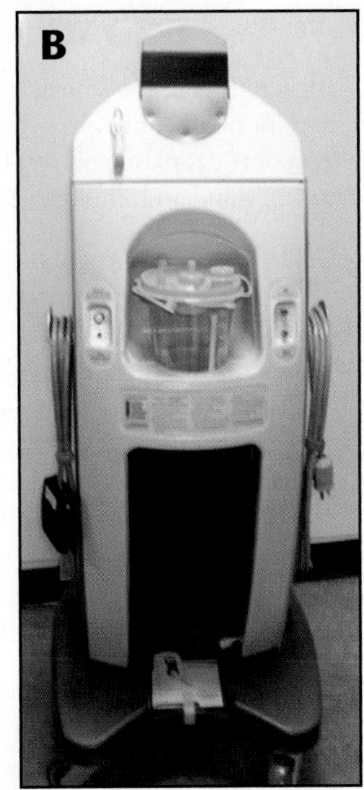

Figure 5-21. Cryotherapy machine front (A) and back (B).

Chapter 5

EGD With Polypectomy

Gastric polyps in the stomach should be removed since the size, distribution, or number of polyps does not reliably differentiate adenomatous from non-neoplastic polyps. Removal may be performed endoscopically using standard hot biopsy forceps or cautery snare techniques.

Equipment

1. Same as for a diagnostic EGD.
2. Biopsy forceps
3. Standard polypectomy snare; looping and clipping devices are also available to assist in hemostasis (Figure 5-22)
4. Bipolar/monopolar electrosurgical cautery unit with grounding pad and cautery probe (Figure 5-23)
5. Tripod grasping forceps or Roth basket (United States Endoscopy Group Inc, Mentor, Ohio) for polyp retrieval (Figures 5-24 and 5-25)
6. Mucus trap (to capture smaller polyps instead of using the tripod grasping forceps)
7. Epinephrine 1:1000 (in a 10-cc syringe mixed with 9 cc of saline for a dilution of 1:10,000) and sclerotherapy needle (the physician may wish to inject the base of the polyp before removal to reduce the risk of bleeding)

Nursing Implications

Preprocedure

- Same as for a diagnostic EGD.
- Give prophylactic antibiotics (if indicated).
- Anticoagulant therapy may be adjusted or discontinued on the advice of the physician.

Intraprocedure

- Patient positioning: Same as for a diagnostic EGD.
- Patient monitoring: Same as for a diagnostic EGD.
- Topical anesthetic: Same as for a diagnostic EGD.
- Additional comfort measures: Same as for a diagnostic EGD.

Postprocedure

- Same as for a diagnostic EGD.

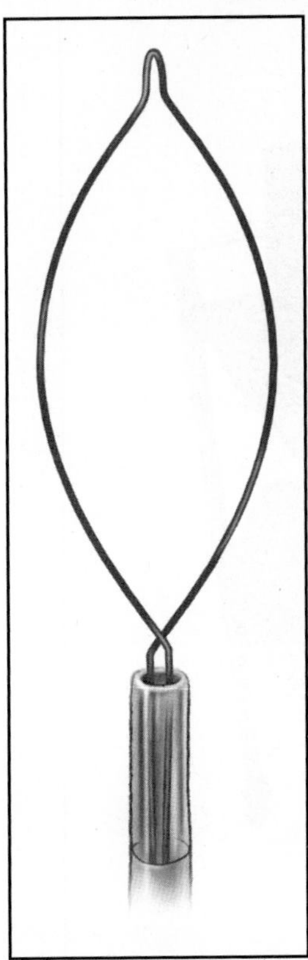

Figure 5-22a. Polypectomy snare.

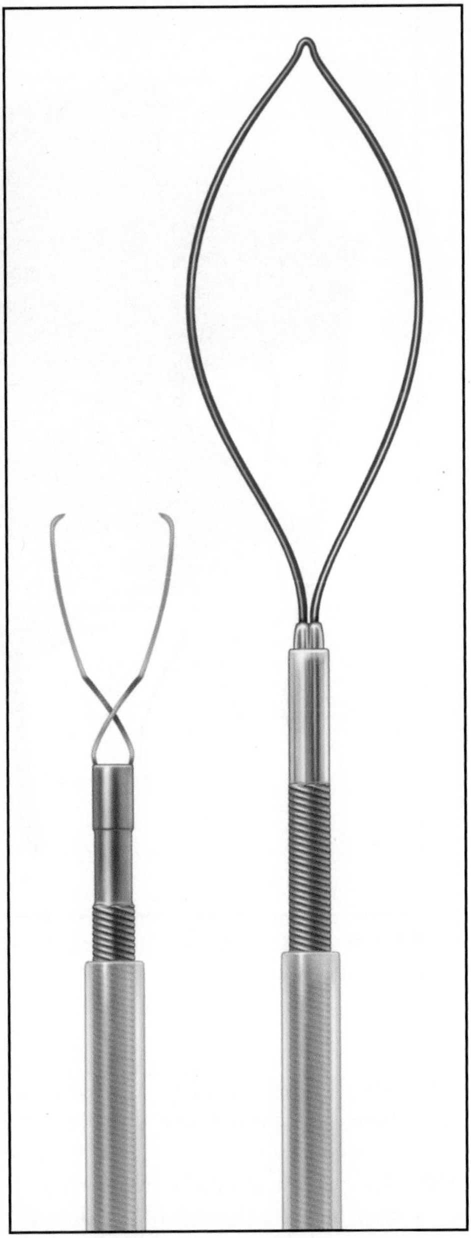

Figure 5-22b. Clipping and snare device.

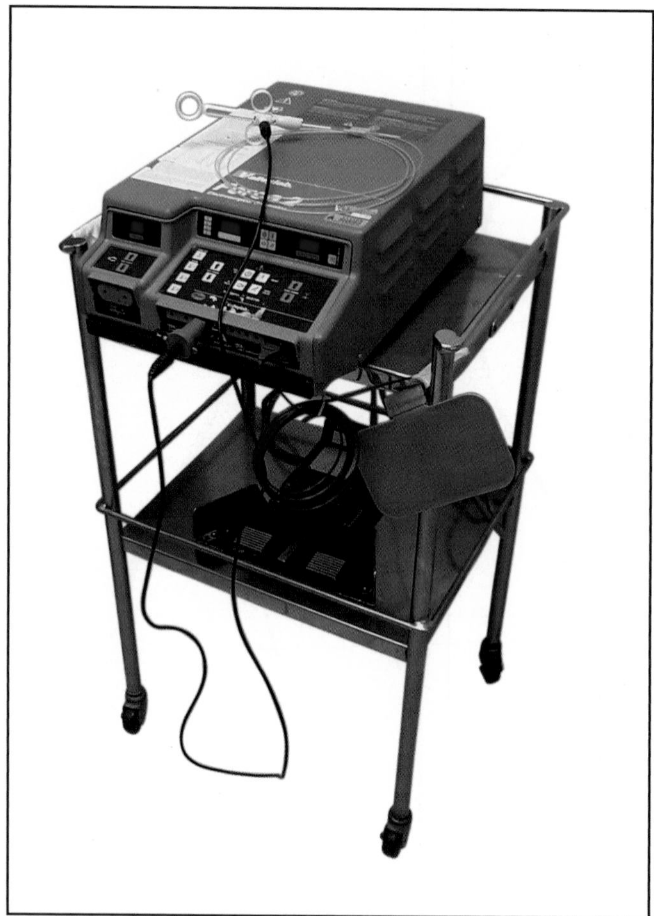

Figure 5-23. Electrosurgical cautery unit with grounding pad and snare.

- The patient should be advised to adhere to a soft diet for 24 hours after polyp removal to prevent mechanical abrasion to the excised area.
- The patient should be instructed to avoid any medications that may increase the risk of bleeding (eg, aspirin) for 1 week after the procedure, on the direction of the physician.

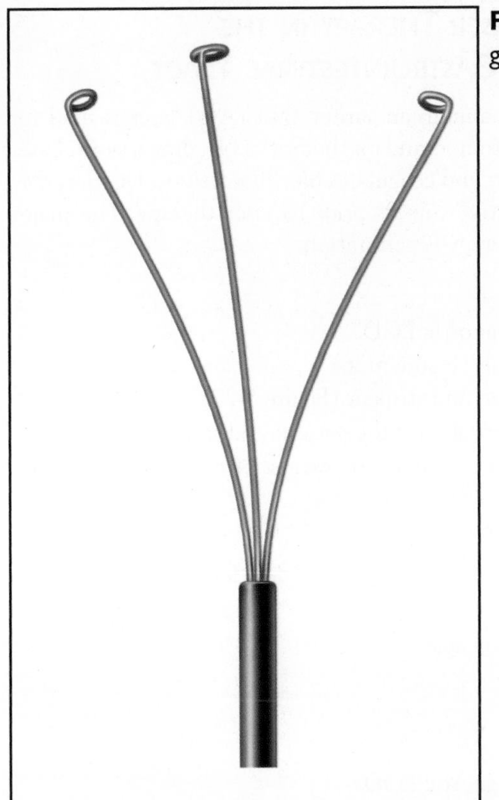

Figure 5-24. Tripod grasping forceps.

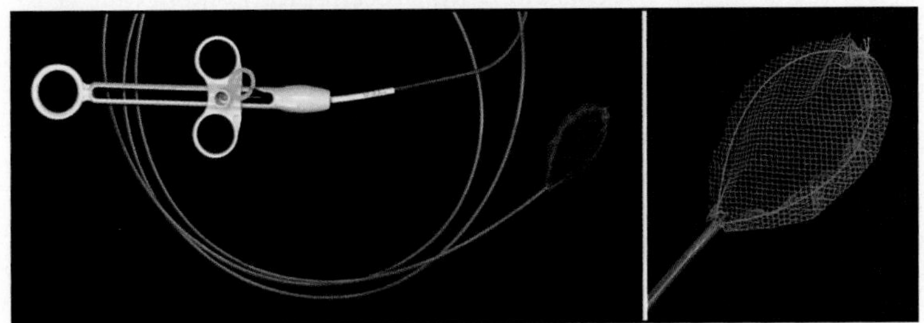

Figure 5-25. Roth basket.

Chapter 5

Laser Therapy in the Upper Gastrointestinal Tract

Neodymium:yttrium-aluminum-garnet (Nd:YAG) laser is used for palliation of malignant tumors and for therapy of bleeding lesions. Laser therapy vaporizes tumors and coagulates bleeding lesions. Dilation may be required for obstructive tumors prior to laser therapy. The major complication of this therapy is perforation.

Equipment

1. Same as for a diagnostic EGD.
2. Nd:YAG laser unit (Figure 5-26)
3. Laser fibers, cutter, and stripper (Figure 5-27)
4. Protective laser goggles for the patient and staff
5. Charcoal filter to eliminate the escape of noxious gases during therapy (Figure 5-28)
6. Laser warning sign

Additional Equipment That May be Needed

1. Polypectomy snare
2. Tripod grasping forceps

Nursing Implications

Preprocedure

- Same as for a diagnostic EGD.
- If the patient is to receive prophylactic antibiotics, it should be done at this time.
- If the patient has coagulopathy, a recent prothrombin time (PT) or partial thromboplastin time (PTT) should be available.
- The patient should have nothing by mouth for 8 hours prior to the procedure except for cases of emergent bleeding.

Intraprocedure

- Patient positioning: Same as for a diagnostic EGD.
- Patient monitoring: Same as for a diagnostic EGD.
- Topical anesthetic: Same as for a diagnostic EGD.
- Additional comfort measures: Same as for a diagnostic EGD.
- Care must be taken to cover the patient's eyes. All personnel in the room should wear goggles as a protective measure, and a laser warning sign should be posted above door to procedure room.

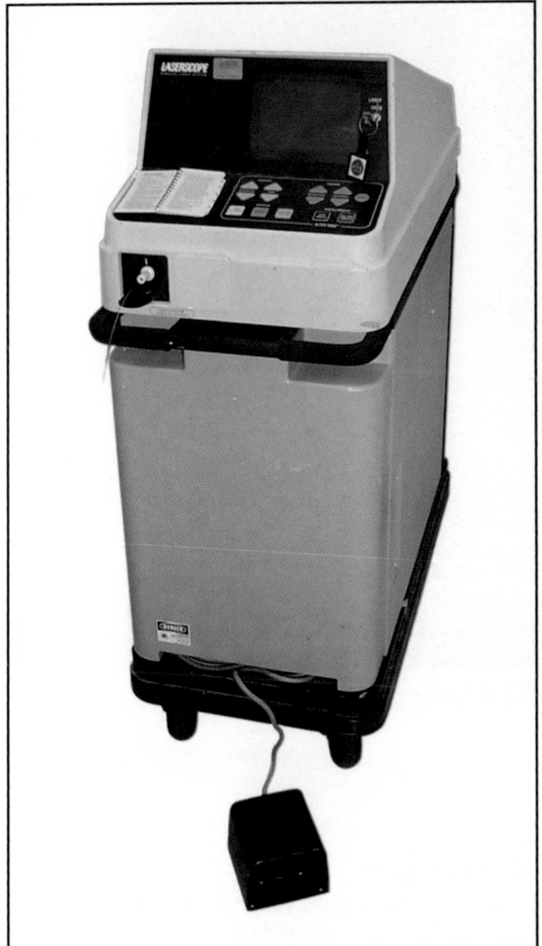

Figure 5-26. Laser unit.

- The tip of the laser fiber may need to be cleaned or revised if deterioration of the tip is noted during the procedure. This may be accomplished by use of the laser cutter and stripper.
- If the fiber is removed from the endoscope at any time during the procedure (usually to clean or cut a new tip), the control panel should be switched to standby position to prevent accidental discharge.

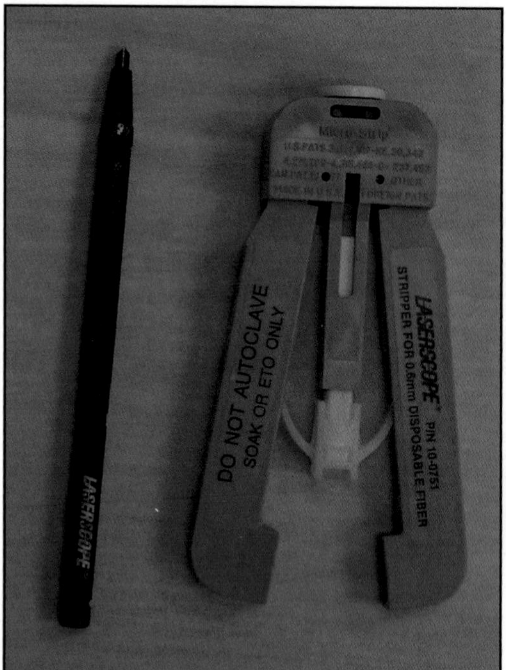

Figure 5-27. Laser cutter and stripper.

Postprocedure

- ❖ Same as for a diagnostic EGD.
- ❖ Diet should consist of clear liquids for the first 24 hours, progressing to full liquids and then to solid foods as tolerated.

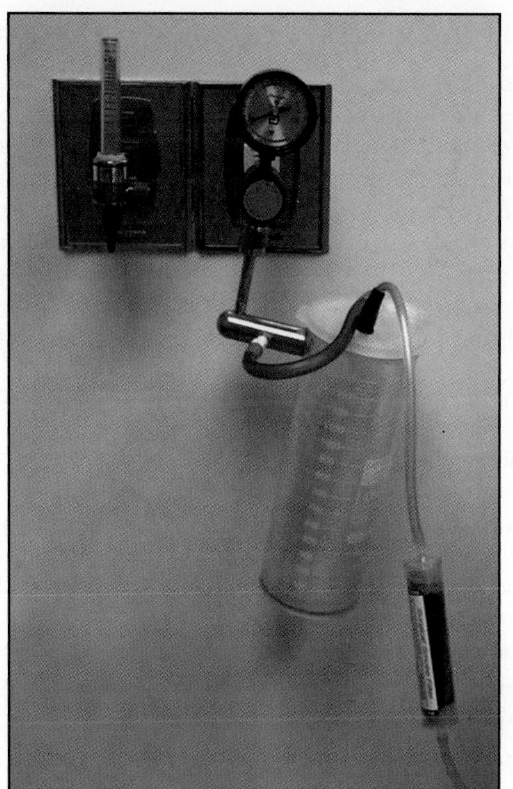

Figure 5-28. Charcoal filter connections.

Chapter 5

EGD With Esophageal Stent Placement

An esophageal stent is an expandable metallic mesh or plastic silicone coated tube used in patients with esophageal cancer for palliative treatment of obstruction or fistula. The stent is usually advanced using fluoroscopic control over a guidewire after the endoscope is withdrawn. Dilation of the obstruction may be necessary before the stent can be placed. The metal mesh-covered stents are normally used for malignant tumors or strictures. The silicone-coated vinyl stents are better suited for benign tumors or strictures. Silicone-coated stents have the advantage of resisting tumor ingrowth and sealing concurrent fistulae.

Equipment (Figure 5-29)

1. Same as for a diagnostic EGD.
2. Hollow polyvinyl dilators and .038-inch diameter guidewire (see Figure 5-8A)
3. Expandable metal stents of assorted lengths: 40 mm, 60 mm, and 90 mm depending on the size of the tumor; silicone-coated stents are available also in multiple lengths and widths.
4. Water-soluble lubricant
5. Fluoroscopy
6. Sclerotherapy needle with water-soluble contrast or topical radiopaque methods

Nursing Implications

Preprocedure

- Same as for a diagnostic EGD.
- Discontinuation of aspirin and nonsteroidal anti-inflammatory drugs (NSAIDs) for 1 week prior to the procedure.
- If the patient is to receive prophylactic antibiotics, it should be done at this time.
- Availability of stent sizes should be ascertained when the procedure is scheduled.
- The patient should be aware that severe gastroesophageal reflux might result if the stent is placed across the gastroesophageal junction.

Intraprocedure

- Patient positioning: Same as for a diagnostic EGD, or the patient may be supine with a 45-degree elevation of the head of the bed to prevent aspiration.

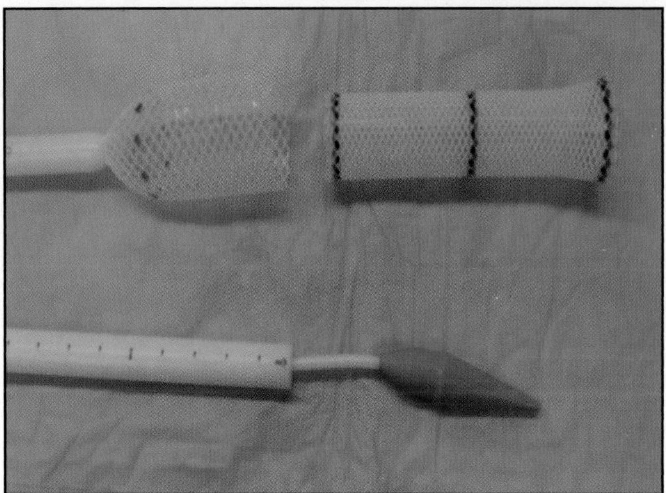

Figure 5-29. Silicone-coated flexible plastic stent.

- ❖ Patient monitoring: Same as for a diagnostic EGD.
- ❖ Topical anesthesia: Same as for a diagnostic EGD.
- ❖ Additional comfort measures: Same as for a diagnostic EGD.
- ❖ The patient may be turned on his or her back to check for proper positioning of the stent, with elevation of the head of the table to reduce aspiration.
- ❖ A second assistant is necessary to aid in equipment management and stent deployment.
- ❖ Fluoroscopy facilitates accurate placement of the stent. Radiopaque markers placed on the patient or contrast injected into the upper and lower borders of the tumor may be used as landmarks for stent placement.
- ❖ Oropharyngeal suctioning is important due to increased secretions (a result of esophageal obstruction) and concomitant risk of aspiration.

Postprocedure

- ❖ Same as for a diagnostic EGD.
- ❖ The patient may complain of chest pain following the procedure from expansion of the stent. The patient should be evaluated

by a physician for chest pain or abdominal pain following the procedure.

- Nutritional consult is necessary for patient education about a modified diet (eg, low fiber, sips of water after each bite).

ENDOSCOPIC ULTRASONOGRAPHY

Endoscopic ultrasonography (EUS) uses high-frequency sound waves to image internal structures. Differing reflection signals are produced when sound waves are projected into the body and reflected, generating an image. EUS displays an image that enables tumor staging and visualization of marginal structures.

EUS may be used for evaluating submucosal lesions, determining their location, and their depth of penetration. EUS may also aid in the evaluation of patients with conditions such as Barrett's esophagus, portal hypertension, chronic pancreatitis, suspected pancreatic neoplasms, and biliary tract disease.

There are several different manufacturers of ultrasound endoscopes. The type of endoscope used is dictated by physician preference. The ultrasound endoscope is relatively fragile. It is important to handle the tip gently. Ultrasound endoscopes should be hung in a closet with the tip encased in a plastic or sponge holder to prevent damage.

EQUIPMENT

1. Ultrasound unit (consisting of monitor, power source, and computer) (Figure 5-30)
2. EUS endoscope:
   a. The radial screening endoscope, used primarily for diagnostic purposes (Figure 5-31)
   b. The linear array endoscope, used for ultrasound-guided biopsies (fine needle biopsy) and to view images in different planes (Figure 5-32)
   c. R-probes are used for obstructive tumors in the esophagus and bile ducts; they employ higher frequencies and are used for very small lesions, giving clearer images.
3. Large water bottle with connecting tubing

NURSING IMPLICATIONS

Preprocedure

- ❖ Same as for a diagnostic EGD.
- ❖ Before placing the balloon on the endoscope tip, the nurse should make certain the balloon water channel is sufficiently purged to prevent the insufflation of large amounts of air.

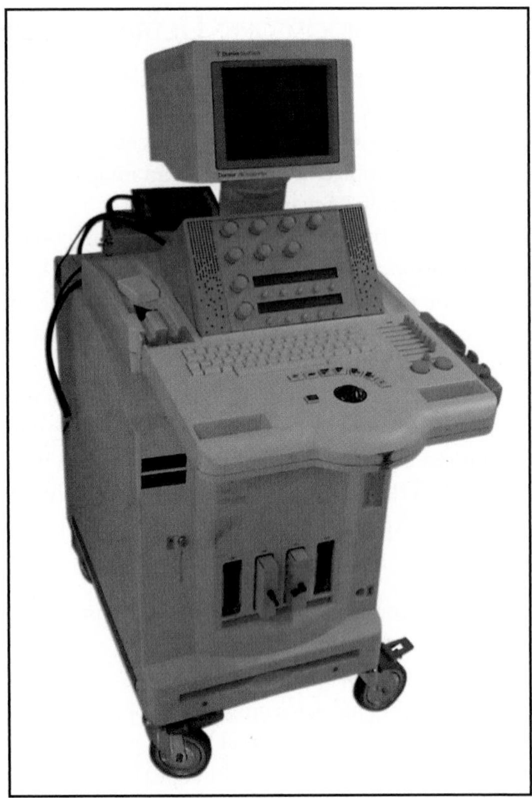

Figure 5-30. EUS unit.

Intraprocedure

- Patient positioning: Same as for a diagnostic EGD.
- Patient monitoring: Same as for a diagnostic EGD.
- Topical anesthesia: Same as for a diagnostic EGD.
- Additional comfort measures: Same as for a diagnostic EGD.
- The procedure may be lengthy; the nurse should keep the patient as comfortable and quiet as possible.

Postprocedure

- Same as for a diagnostic EGD.

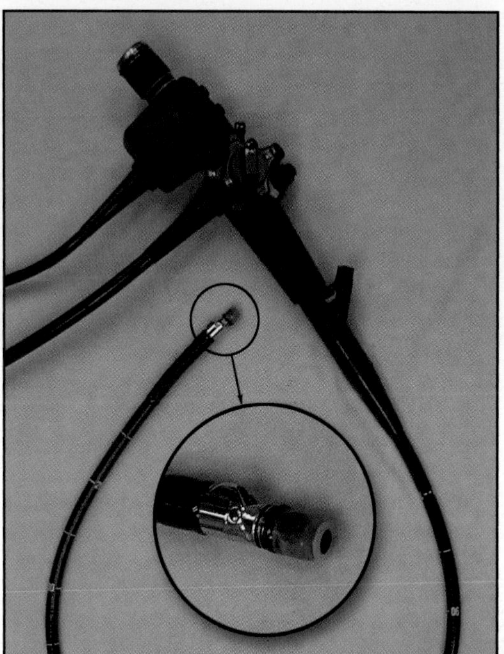

Figure 5-31. EUS upper endoscope.

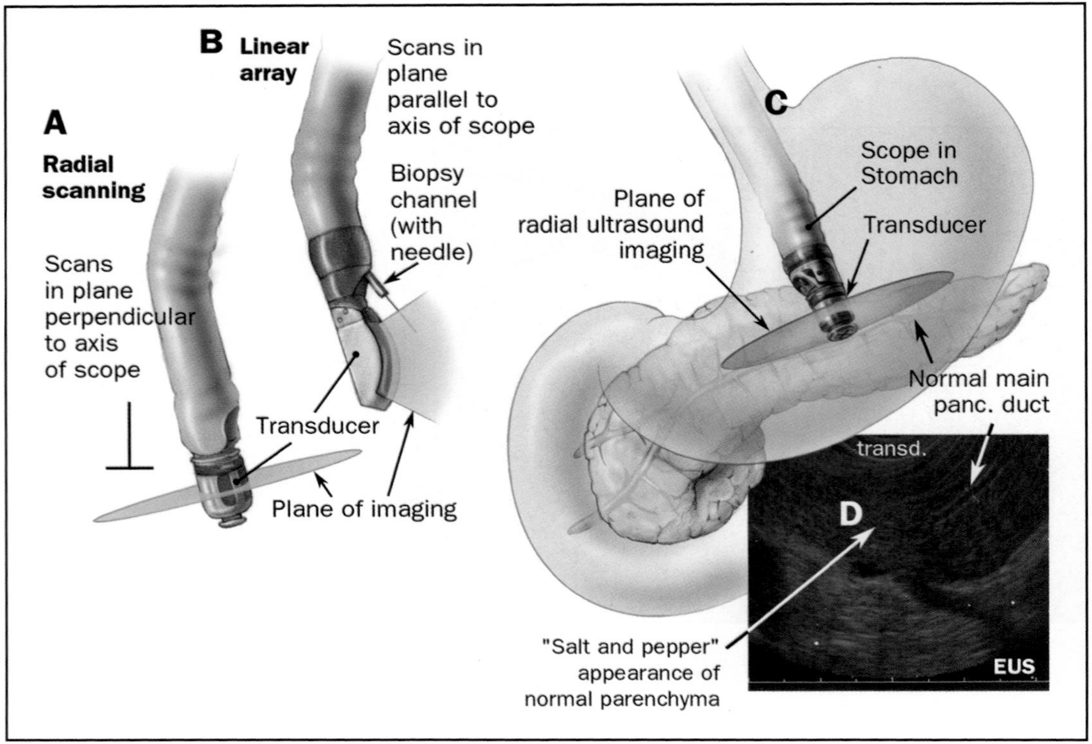

Figure 5-32. Radial (A) and linear (B) array ultrasound endoscopes.

EUS With Fine Needle Aspiration

Fine needle aspiration (FNA) allows the physician to obtain cells for cytopathological examination. First, EUS locates the lesion. Then, a EUS needle is passed through the biopsy channel of the endoscope and into the lesion to aspirate cells.

Equipment

1. Same as for EUS.
2. FNA needle (Figure 5-33)
3. Sheath
4. Stylet
5. 100 cc of sterile normal saline irrigating solution
6. 10-cc luer-lock syringe
7. Clear slides
8. 95% alcohol

Nursing Implications

Preprocedure

- Same as for a diagnostic EGD.
- Discontinuation of aspirin and NSAIDs for 1 week prior to the procedure.
- If the patient is to receive prophylactic antibiotics, it should be done at this time.
- If the patient has been on anticoagulant therapy, a recent PT and PTT should be available.
- A cytopathologist should be available at the time of EUS to prepare the slides for reading and interpretation.

Intraprocedure

- Same as for EUS.
- An assistant is required for specimen collection while the nurse monitors sedation, patient comfort, and vital signs.
- An increased procedure time may be necessary since multiple (one to eight) passes may be required before an adequate number of cells are obtained.

Postprocedure

- Same as for EUS.

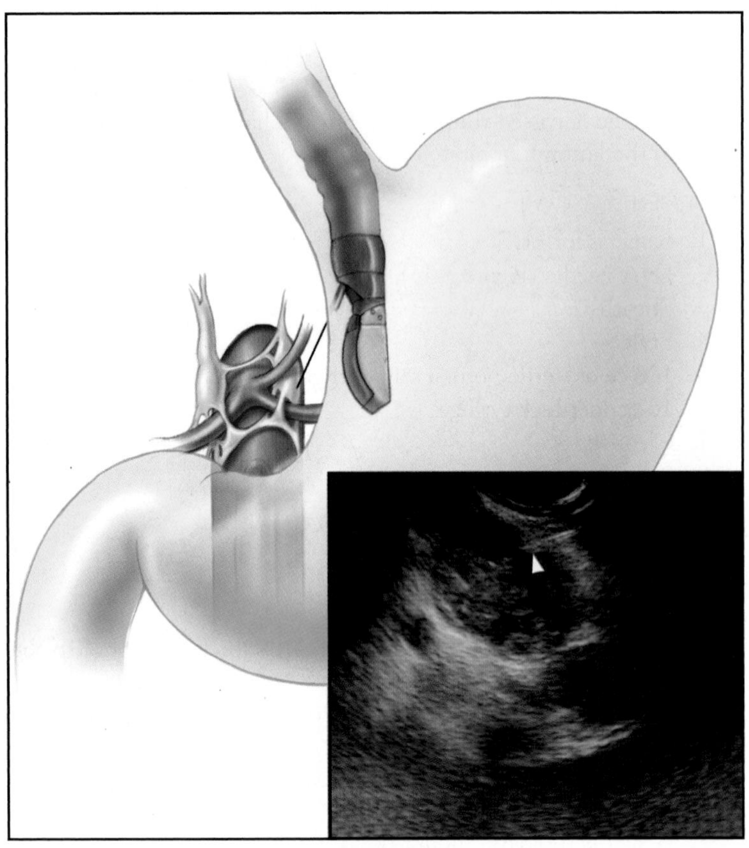

Figure 5-33. EUS endoscope with FNA.

Percutaneous Endoscopic Gastrostomy Tube Placement

Percutaneous endoscopic gastrostomy (PEG) refers to the endoscopic placement of a gastric feeding tube. The most common indication for PEG placement is failure of oral feedings. Patients with swallowing problems (stroke, severe psychomotor retardation, birth asphyxia, progressive degenerative diseases, neurologic neoplasm, or trauma) and patients with esophageal obstruction (oropharyngeal and esophageal carcinoma) may benefit from PEG placement. A PEG tube may be used to deliver unpalatable medications and supplemental feedings in children with inflammatory bowel disease. PEGs are also used in patients for gastric decompression from chronic bowel obstruction or gastric atony and as a conduit for bile replacement when internal drainage is not feasible.

Equipment

1. Upper endoscope
2. Bite block
3. Topical anesthesia
4. PEG kit: contains Betadine swabs (Purdue Frederick, Norwalk, Conn), sterile 4x4 pads, a vial of lidocaine for injection, a 5-cc syringe with 25-g needle, 20-g 1.5-inch needle, a snare (pediatric endoscopes require pediatric snares), a scalpel, a 20-Fr gastrostomy tube with bumper and end plug, a fenestrated sterile drape, lubricant, and antibiotic ointment. Some kits also provide a hemostat and scissor.

Nursing Implications

Preprocedure

- Same as for a diagnostic EGD.
- The physician may prescribe cephalosporin to be given 1 hour prior to the procedure. This has been shown to significantly reduce infectious complications.
- The patient or responsible caretaker should receive instructions regarding administration of tube feedings and care of the PEG.
- The room should be easily darkened to facilitate transillumination of the abdominal wall.

Intraprocedure (Figure 5-34)

- Patient positioning:
  1. The patient is usually placed supine with the head and chest elevated to about 45 degrees to prevent aspiration. This also exposes the abdominal area for ease of tube placement. When surveying the abdomen for proper tube placement, location of surgical scars should be noted. Scarred areas may make tube placement difficult.
- Patient monitoring: Same as for a diagnostic EGD.
- Topical anesthesia: Same as for a diagnostic EGD.
- Frequent suctioning is needed for increased oral secretions.
- Strict aseptic technique should be observed during the procedure.
- The nurse may assist the physician in transillumination (visualizing the endoscope light through the abdomen) to determine the site for PEG placement.
- Additional comfort measures: Same as for a diagnostic EGD.
- After the gastric tube is in place and the bumper is applied, care must be taken to ensure that there is no excess traction. This excess traction may cause a necrotizing fasciitis (necrosis of tissue under and around the bumper because of ischemia). Antibiotic ointment and a dry dressing may be applied to the wound site.

Postprocedure

- Same as for a diagnostic EGD.
- The patient may remain on his or her back with the head elevated or may lie on his or her side until fully awake.
- Dietary instructions; instructions regarding signs and symptoms of bleeding, perforation, infection; and follow-up should be given to the patient before he or she leaves the unit.
- The patient may be discharged with instructions regarding care of the tube and feeding administration.

Care of the PEG and Feeding Tubes

- The dressing should be checked every 4 hours for the first 24 hours for purulent or bloody discharge.
- The area around the tube may be cleansed with soap and water. A clean, dry dressing may be reapplied until the incision is

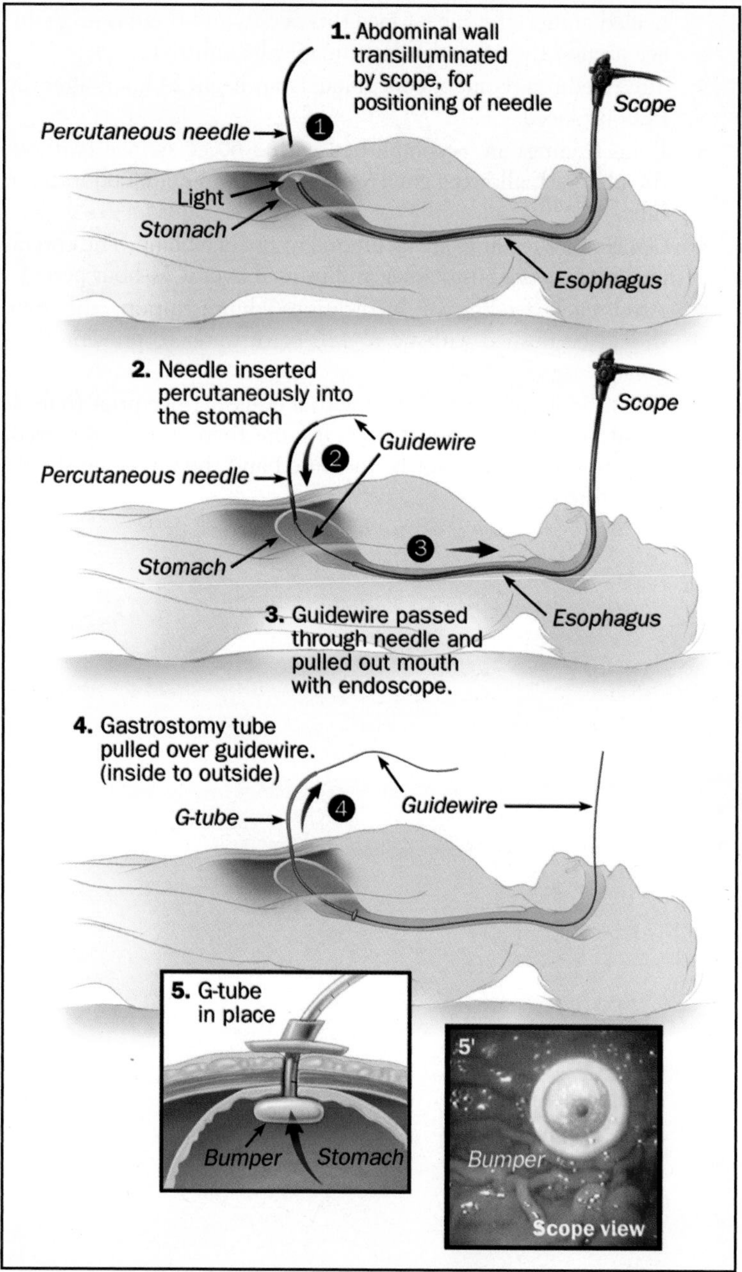

Figure 5-34. Steps of PEG placement.

healed around the tube. Once this occurs and there is no drainage around the tube, the dressing may be omitted.

- Tube feedings (bolus or continuous) may begin 24 hours after the PEG is placed.
- Bolus feedings are accomplished with a 60 cc syringe (without the plunger), allowing gravity to deliver the liquid food into the tube.
- Continuous feedings are facilitated by use of a pump. The enteral feeding is poured into a bag and infused over a 24-hour period.
- After each feeding or medication administration, the tube should be flushed with 60 to 120 cc of water to prevent clogging.
- The tube should be aspirated with a 60-cc syringe prior to feedings to check for residual food. If more than 50 cc is removed, then feeding should not be instituted and the physician should be notified.

Percutaneous Endoscopic Jejunostomy Tube Placement

Percutaneous endoscopic jejunostomy (PEJ) refers to the endoscopic placement of a feeding tube in the jejunum. This procedure is performed in patients with abnormal gastric emptying or severe gastroesophageal reflux with aspiration.

Equipment

1. An existing PEG tube
2. Same as for a diagnostic EGD.
3. Upper endoscope or pediatric endoscope
4. PEJ kit contains the adapter to fit into the PEG tube, a 12-Fr (French) PEJ tube, and a PEJ tube end plug (depending upon the brand, contents of the kit may differ slightly).
5. Biopsy or special grasping forceps
6. Syringe (10 to 20 cc) to flush the tube with water after insertion to determine patency.

Nursing Implications

Preprocedure

- Same as for a diagnostic EGD.
- Intravenous cephalosporin may be prescribed if PEG is performed prior to PEJ.
- Review discharge instructions with the patient and family before sedation. The instructions should also include care of a PEG/PEJ and feeding administration.

Intraprocedure

- Patient positioning: Same as for PEG placement.
- Patient monitoring: Same as for PEG placement.
- Topical anesthetic: Same as for PEG placement.
- Additional comfort measures: Same as for PEG placement.
- During the EGD, the physician should shorten the gastric tube to the desired length. The jejunal tube is threaded into the stomach through the PEG tube until the physician can grasp the tip using biopsy or special grasping forceps.
- The tube is then positioned into the jejunum.

- The nurse must be careful not to thread the PEJ tube (J-tube) through the PEG tube (G-tube) too quickly, as it will loop in the stomach and prevent proper placement.
- Once the physician determines that proper placement is achieved, the endoscope is carefully withdrawn.
- The J-tube is flushed with water to ensure patency and the guidewire is removed.

Postprocedure

- Same as for PEG placement.

Care of the PEG/PEJ and Tube Feeding

- It is important to flush the tube with 60 to 100 cc of water after every use to prevent clogging.
- Feeding may begin immediately after insertion.
- Depending on the type of G-tube placed, a wound dressing may not be necessary. Cleaning the area with soap and water and applying an antibiotic ointment is sufficient.
- The patient should be instructed to notify the physician if the G-tube site becomes inflamed, painful, or has a purulent discharge.

Endoscopic Nasoenteric Tube Placement

Endoscopic nasoenteric tube placement refers to endoscopic placement of a nasal tube into the duodenum for short-term therapy for feeding and suctioning. Depending upon the tube type, it may have a gastric port for drainage or lavage. Drawbacks of the nasoenteric tube include erosion of the nasal cartilage, esophagitis, aspiration, and patient discomfort.

Equipment

1. Upper endoscope
2. Bite block
3. Topical anesthetic
4. Nasoenteric tube kit (Figure 5-35) contains one nasoenteric tube and guidewire, stylet for stiffening, plug, and adhesive fastener.
5. Water-soluble lubricant
6. Biopsy forceps

Nursing Implications

Preprocedure

- Same as for a diagnostic EGD.
- Review discharge instructions, including care of the nasoenteric tube and tube feedings, with the patient or caregiver before sedation.

Intraprocedure

- Patient positioning:
  1. Same as for PEG tube placement.
  2. Transillumination of the abdomen is not necessary since placement is accomplished nasally.
- Patient monitoring: Same as for PEG tube placement.
- Topical anesthetic: Same as for a diagnostic EGD.
- The nasoenteric tube is placed into the nose before or after the endoscope has already been passed into the stomach. The tube needs to be well-lubricated with anesthetic jelly or water-soluble lubricant.
- The physician grasps the string attached to the tube with biopsy forceps and positions it into the second portion of the duodenum (fully extending the tube).

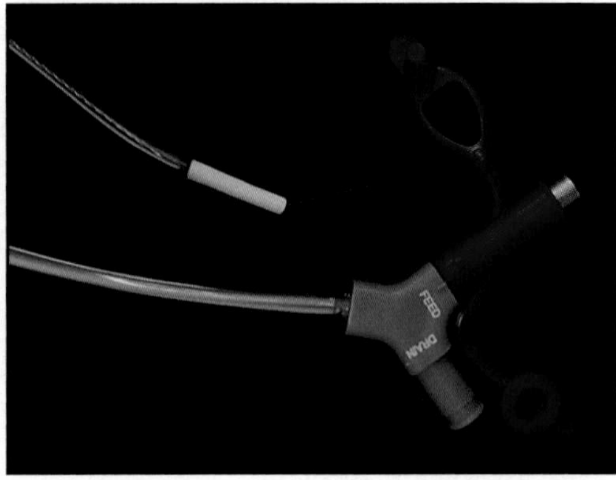

Figure 5-35. Naso-enteric tube kit.

- The endoscope should be carefully removed and the tube flushed with water to ensure patency.
- The guidewire should be removed and the tube taped securely to the nose.
- Additional comfort measures: Care must be taken not to pull the tube too close to the inside wall of the nostril, as this may cause ulceration.

Photodynamic Therapy

Photodynamic therapy (PDT) refers to the use of photosensitizing light to treat premalignant and malignant conditions, including those of the gastrointestinal tract. It requires the intravenous administration of a photosensitizing drug (porfimer sodium; Photofrin, QLT PhotoTherapeutics, Vancouver, BC) and the endoscopic application of low-level laser light to selectively destroy dysplastic tissue. Forty to 50 hours after the injection of Photofrin, upper endoscopy is performed. A laser fiber inserted through the biopsy channel of the endoscope is directed to selectively destroy cancer cells while limiting damage to surrounding tissue. The course of treatment may require several applications (Figure 5-36).

Equipment for Photofrin Injection

1. Intravenous supplies (angiocatheter, heparin lock)
2. Scale to measure patient's weight to calculate drug dosage
3. Photofrin
4. Towel (to protect the injection site from light)

Nursing Implications for Photofrin Injection

Preprocedure

- ❖ Verify allergies.
- ❖ Document vital signs and oxygen saturation.
- ❖ Make sure the patient has an understanding of the adverse effects of Photofrin, including light sensitivity.
- ❖ Check for appropriate protective clothing to keep the patient completely shielded from the sun.
- ❖ Insert an intravenous catheter with heparin lock adapter.
- ❖ Weigh the patient.
- ❖ The physician should obtain an informed consent from the patient or responsible adult.

Intraprocedure

- ❖ Secure the medication and verify the calculation of dosage with another nurse.
- ❖ Keep the medication covered and protected from light (the drug is usually dispensed in a syringe covered with an aluminum foil or light-shielding brown cover).

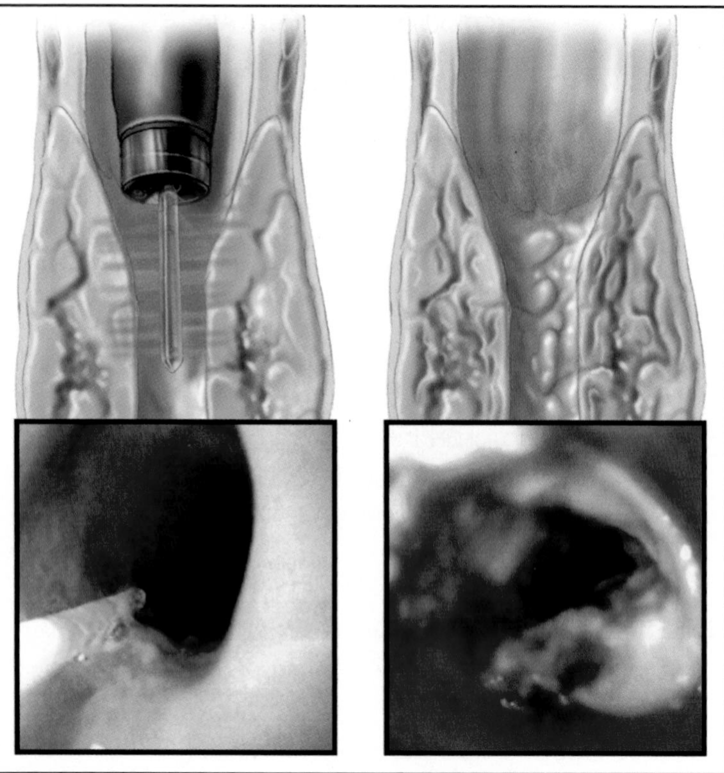

Figure 5-36. Endoscopic technique of light application with subsequent tumor destruction.

- While administering the drug through the IV tubing, care must be taken to cover the tubing with a towel.
- The standard dose of Photofrin is 2 mg/kg administered over 3 to 5 minutes. Always check the Photofrin package insert for precautions, contraindications, and recommended dosage prior to administration.

Postprocedure

- The patient should remain in the recovery room for at least 30 minutes to watch for any untoward drug reactions.

- ❖ Upon patient discharge, the nurse should verify the patient is wearing protective clothing. The possible adverse effects of Photofrin may occur for up to 1 month. After this period of time, exposure to sunlight should be gradual.
- ❖ Patients should be advised to call their physician with signs of respiratory distress, itching, or anaphylaxis.
- ❖ The importance of staying well-hydrated (which may be difficult because of concomitant swallowing difficulties) should be emphasized to the patient. Clear- to full-liquid diet is usually necessary throughout the treatment.

Equipment for PDT Treatment (Figure 5-37)

1. Endoscope
2. Bite block
3. Topical anesthetic
4. Water bottle
5. 630 PDT Laser
6. Delivery fiber
7. Inner cuvette for calibration
8. Safety glasses for patient and staff
9. Laser "Warning" sign for entrance into procedure room

Nursing Implications for PDT Treatment

Preprocedure

- ❖ Same as for a diagnostic EGD.
- ❖ The patient should be instructed about the following:
  1. Photosensitivity precautions (eg, avoiding direct sunlight, wearing appropriate clothing and eye coverings)
  2. Importance of taking prescribed pain medications as necessary
  3. Importance of adequate hydration
  4. Importance of follow-up care

Intraprocedure

- ❖ Patient positioning: Same as for a diagnostic EGD.
- ❖ Patient monitoring: Same as for a diagnostic EGD.
- ❖ Topical anesthetic: Same as for a diagnostic EGD.
- ❖ Follow the manufacturer's instructions for setting up the 630 PDT Laser.

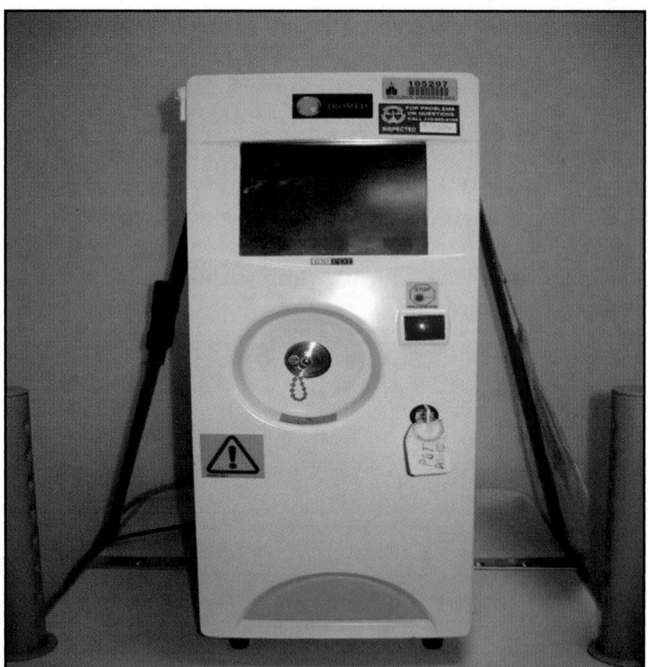

Figure 5-37. PDT module.

- ❖ Provide safety glasses for all staff and patient.
- ❖ Additional comfort measures: Same as for a diagnostic EGD.

Postprocedure

- ❖ Same as for a diagnostic EGD.
- ❖ Discharge patients with instructions regarding protective clothing, diet (clear- to full-liquid diet), prescriptions for pain, a premixed solution consisting of an antacid and antihistamine for throat discomfort, antiemetics, and a proton-pump inhibitor.
- ❖ Home health care referral.

Botulinum Toxin Injection in the Upper Gastrointestinal Tract

Botulinum toxin is a potent neuromuscular blocker. It is used in the upper gastrointestinal tract to relax smooth muscle. In the last decade its use has expanded to include smooth muscle disorders such as achalasia, diffuse esophageal spasm, dysphagia from nonspecific esophageal motility disorders, isolated hypertension of the lower esophageal sphincter, sphincter of Oddi dysfunction, and oropharyngeal dysphagia.

Equipment

1. Same as for a diagnostic EGD.
2. Sclerotherapy needle
3. Vial of botulinum toxin (100 units)
4. 10-cc syringe for botulinum toxin and 3-cc syringe for saline to flush the toxin from the sclerotherapy needle.

Nursing Implications

Preprocedure

- Same as for a diagnostic EGD.
- Procedure for preparation of botulinum toxin:
  1. Keep vial frozen until ready to use.
  2. Check with physician as to the concentration ofbotulinum toxin and add appropriate volume of normal saline to the vial,, taking care not to cause bubbles, as air denatures the toxin.
  3. Do not agitate the vial violently, as this causes denaturization of the mixture.
  4. Draw up the botulinum toxin solution into a 10-cc syringe.
  5. Flush the solution through a standard sclerotherapy needle; this uses about 1.8 cc of the solution.
  6. The physician may direct the nurse to inject incremental doses into the targeted area (Figure 5-38).

Intraprocedure

- Patient positioning: Same as for a diagnostic EGD.
- Patient monitoring: Same as for a diagnostic EGD.
- Topical anesthetic: Same as for a diagnostic EGD.
- It is necessary to use a 3-cc syringe filled with saline to flush the remaining toxin.

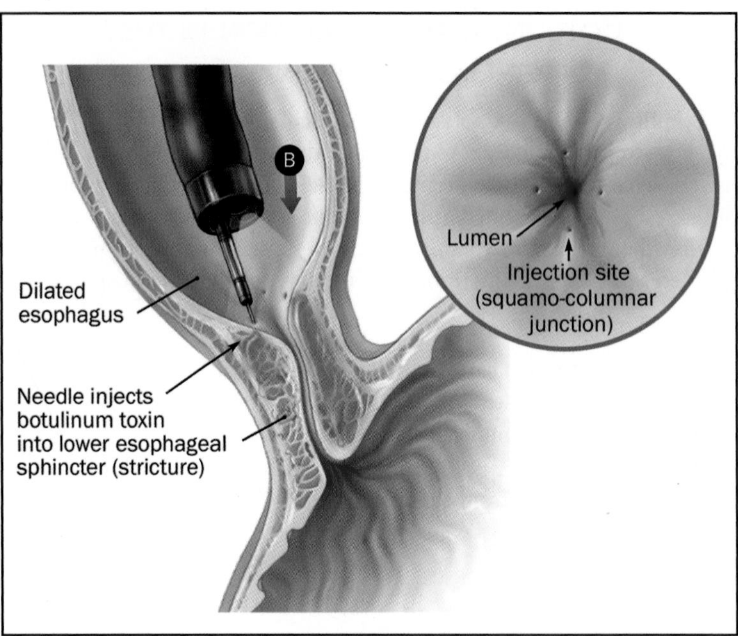

Figure 5-38. Endoscopic technique of botulinum toxin injection into the lower esophageal sphincter.

- ❖ Additional comfort measures: Same as for a diagnostic EGD.
- ❖ There are no special disposal instructions when using botulinum toxin.
- ❖ Needle and glass vial disposal should be performed in the usual manner in accordance with hospital waste policy.

Postprocedure

- ❖ Same as for a diagnostic EGD.
- ❖ Systemic complications are rare but include transient skin rash.
- ❖ Local side effects may be related to the targeted sphincter or organ (eg, esophageal reflux as a result of lowering esophageal pressure).

Chromoendoscopy

Chromoendoscopy (Figure 5-39) involves the topical application of dyes to alter tissue appearance and improve localization, characterization, and diagnosis of dysplastic mucosal lesions (such as Barrett's esophagus). Chromoendoscopy usually adds 5 to 10 minutes to the endoscopic procedure.

Lugol's solution stains normal squamous cells of the esophagus brownish-black or greenish-brown within moments and gradually fades in a couple of hours. Abnormal cells do not stain. The technique is useful to detect high-grade dysplasia and early squamous cell cancers of the esophagus.

Methylene blue selectively stains specialized columnar epithelium in patients with Barrett's esophagus. Light or absent blue staining is associated with high-grade dysplasia or cancer.

Acetic acid (vinegar) spray is used as a mucolytic agent and administered prior to application of the dye to enhance staining.

Equipment

1. Spray catheter
2. Two 60-cc syringes
3. 20-cc syringe
4. 30 cc of mucolytic solution (when using methylene blue)
5. 10 cc of methylene blue
6. 10 cc of 5% Lugol's solution (if requested)
7. 10 cc of 5% acetic acid diluted with 10 cc of normal saline
8. Therapeutic endoscope (if large biopsies are to be obtained)
9. Jumbo biopsy forceps

Nursing Implications

Preprocedure

- ❖ Same as for a diagnostic EGD.
- ❖ A recent PT and PTT should be available.
- ❖ If the patient is to receive prophylactic antibiotics, it should be done at this time.

Intraprocedure

- ❖ Patient positioning: Same as for a diagnostic EGD.
- ❖ Patient monitoring: Same as for a diagnostic EGD.

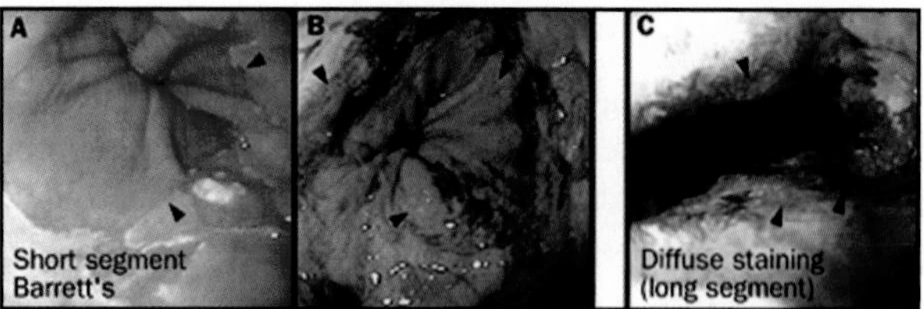

Figure 5-39. Chromoendoscopy (mucosa).

- Topical anesthesia: Same as for a diagnostic EGD.
- Additional comfort measures:
  1. Use a new biopsy cap to prevent dye from leaking out.
  2. Elevate the head of the bed to 30 degrees in addition to frequent oral suctioning to prevent aspiration.
- Acetic acid preparation:
  1. Put 10 cc 5% acetic acid mixed with 10cc normal saline in a 20 cc syringe.
  2. Insert spray catheter through the biopsy channel of the endoscope and spray the affected area at physician's command.
- Methylene blue preparation procedure:
  1. Mix 30 cc of mucolytic solution with 30 cc of water in a 60-cc syringe.
  2. Mix 10 cc of methylene blue with 10 cc of water in a 20-cc syringe.
  3. Insert spray catheter through the biopsy channel of the endoscope.
- When instructed by the physician, spray the affected area with mucolytic solution (Mucomyst, AstraZeneca, Wilmington, Del) and wait 2 minutes. When instructed by the physician, spray methylene blue and wait 2 minutes.
- Flush area with 60 cc or more of water until the area is cleared.
- Assist the physician with biopsies.
- After the procedure, flush the endoscope with 50 to 100 cc of water until clear of dye.
- Lugol's solution preparation procedure:
  1. Mix 30 cc of 5% Lugol's solution with 30 cc of water in a 60-cc syringe.

2. Insert spray catheter through the biopsy channel of the endoscope.
3. Spray the affected area.
4. After the procedure, flush the endoscope with 50 to 100 cc of water until clear of dye.

Postprocedure

- Same as for a diagnostic EGD.
- It should be explained to the patient that his or her stools may be darker for up to 2 weeks due to the blue dye.

Chapter 5

EGD WITH NARROW BAND IMAGING

Narrow band imaging (NBI) is a lighting system based on narrowing the bandwidth of transmitted light using optical filters. This allows fewer wavelengths of light within the RGB (red, green blue) spectrum to pass through the optical fibers of the endoscope. Blue light, a shorter wavelength, penetrates only the superficial layers, improving resolution. This technology is useful in the early detection of dysplasia of Barrett's esophagus.

EQUIPMENT

1. Same as for diagnostic EGD except for the narrow band imaging endoscope (Olympus GIFQ240Z; Olympus America, Center Valley, PA) (Figure 5-40).
2. Spray catheter
3. 20 cc syringe
4. 10 cc normal saline
5. 10 cc 5% acetic acid

EUS

NURSING IMPLICATIONS

Preprocedure

- Same as for diagnostic EGD.

Intraprocedure

- Same as for diagnostic EGD.
- Acetic acid preparation:
    1. Put 10 cc 5% acetic acid mixed with 10 cc normal saline in a 20 cc syringe.
    2. Insert spray catheter through the biopsy channel of the endoscope and spray the affected area as directed by the physician.

Postprocedure

- Same as for diagnostic EGD.

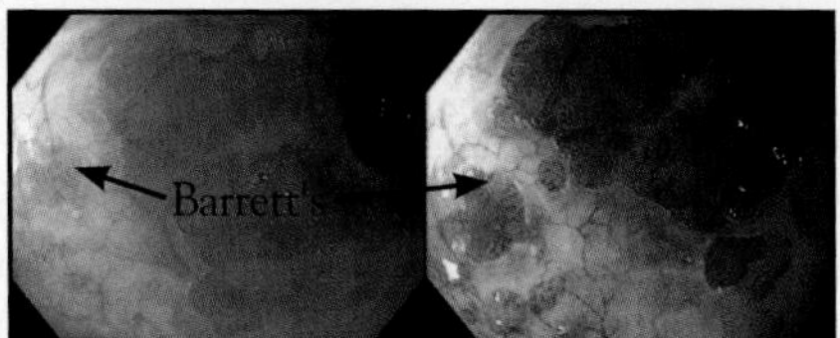

Figure 5-40. Narrow band imaging

Chapter 5

CONFOCAL LASER ENDOMICROSCOPY

Confocal laser endomicroscopy (CLE) is an endoscopic procedure that enables the surface of the intestinal or gastric mucosa to be examined microscopically in vivo during the endoscopy. This is accomplished by the integration of a small confocal microscope (Figure 5-41) at the distal tip of a conventional endoscope, allowing quantitative measurements of surface mucosa in both lateral and vertical dimensions. Cellular, vascular and connective structures can be seen in detail with a maximum magnifying power of 1000X. Using point scanning laser analysis, the physician is able to have a real time diagnosis of different GI diagnoses such as Barrett's Esophagus, helicobacter pylori gastritis, colon cancer and ulcerative colitis screening and early gastric cancer.

EQUIPMENT

1. Set up confocal endoscope and processors according to manufacture's instructions (Pentax EC-3870CIK; Pentax Medical Company, Montvale, NJ).
2. Fluorescein 5 mg, contrast agent, frequently used in ophthalmology, is injected intravenously to enhance the resolution of the endomicroscopic image.
3. 5 cc syringe
4. Spray catheter

NURSING IMPLICATIONS

Preprocedure

- ❖ Same as for diagnostic EGD.
- ❖ Assess patient for allergies.
- ❖ Instruct patient on side effects of fluorescein; yellow skin and eyes for several hours after the procedure, contact lenses should not be worn until the following day, and urine may be bright orange or yellow in color for 12 to 15 hours after the injection of the fluorescein.

Intraprocedure

- ❖ Same as for diagnostic EGD.

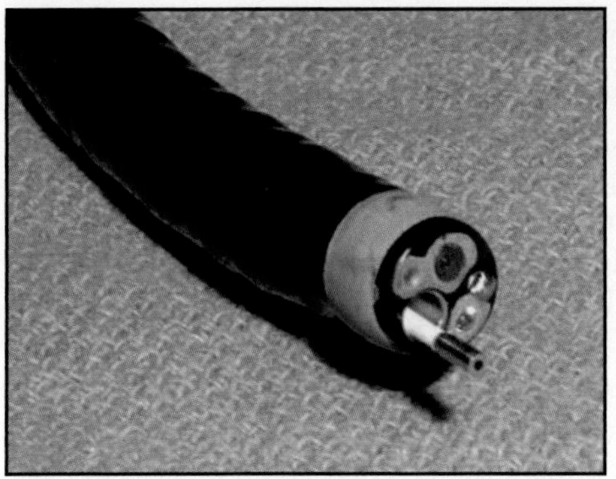

Figure 5-41. Confocal scope.

- ❖ Prepare fluorescein 5 mg to be given slowly via IV push.
- ❖ Monitor patient for adverse side effects such as:

Common

1. Cardiovascular: Hypotension, syncope
2. Gastrointestinal: Drug-induced gastrointestinal disturbance such as nausea, altered taste sense, and vomiting
3. Immunologic: Generalized pruritus, hives
4. Neurologic: Headache
5. Respiratory: Bronchospasm

Serious

1. Cardiovascular: Arterial ischemia, cardiac arrest, shock (Severe)
2. Dermatologic: Injection site; thrombophlebitis

Immunologic: Anaphylaxis

Neurologic: Seizure

Postprocedure

- ❖ Same as for diagnostic EGD.

Chapter 5

Endoscopic Mucosal Resection

Endoscopic mucosal resection (EMR) refers to endoscopic removal of the gastrointestinal mucosa. This technique is used to treat patients with dysplasia and early superficial cancer confined to the mucosa. The most common techniques of EMR are strip biopsy, double snare polypectomy, resection with saline and epinephrine, and resection using a cap and the Cook Medical Duette Mucosectomy (Cook Medical Inc., Bloomington, IN).

The following is an abbreviated explanation of each method:

- Strip biopsy: This method utilizes a double-channel endoscope with grasping forceps and a snare. The lesion border is marked with electrocautery. Using a sclerotherapy needle, saline is injected into the submucosa below the lesion, causing separation from the muscle layer and protrusion. Grasping forceps are then passed through the loop of a snare to elevate the tissue. The mucosa surrounding the lesion is then grasped and strangulated with the snare. The resection is accomplished with snare electrocautery (Figure 5-42).
- Double-snare polypectomy: This method uses a double-channel endoscope with two snares and is suitable for protruding lesions. The first snare is used to grasp and lift the lesion from the muscle layer while the second is used to complete the resection with electrocautery (Figure 5-43).
- Endoscopic resection with injection of concentrated saline and epinephrine: This method is performed with a double-channel endoscope. The lesion borders are marked with cautery, and a highly concentrated saline and epinephrine solution is injected (15 to 20 cc) into the submucosal layer. This causes the area to swell, making the markings more visible. A high-frequency scalpel is used to excise the lesion to the level of the submucosa. The mucosa is lifted, trapped with a snare, and resected by electrocautery (Figure 5-44).
- Endoscopic resection by clear cap: This method utilizes a clear cap equipped with a prelooped snare. After its insertion, the cap is placed on the lesion and the mucosa is aspirated into the cap. The mucosa is caught and strangulated by the snare and resected by electrocautery. The specimen is retained in the cap for histological examination (Figure 5-45).

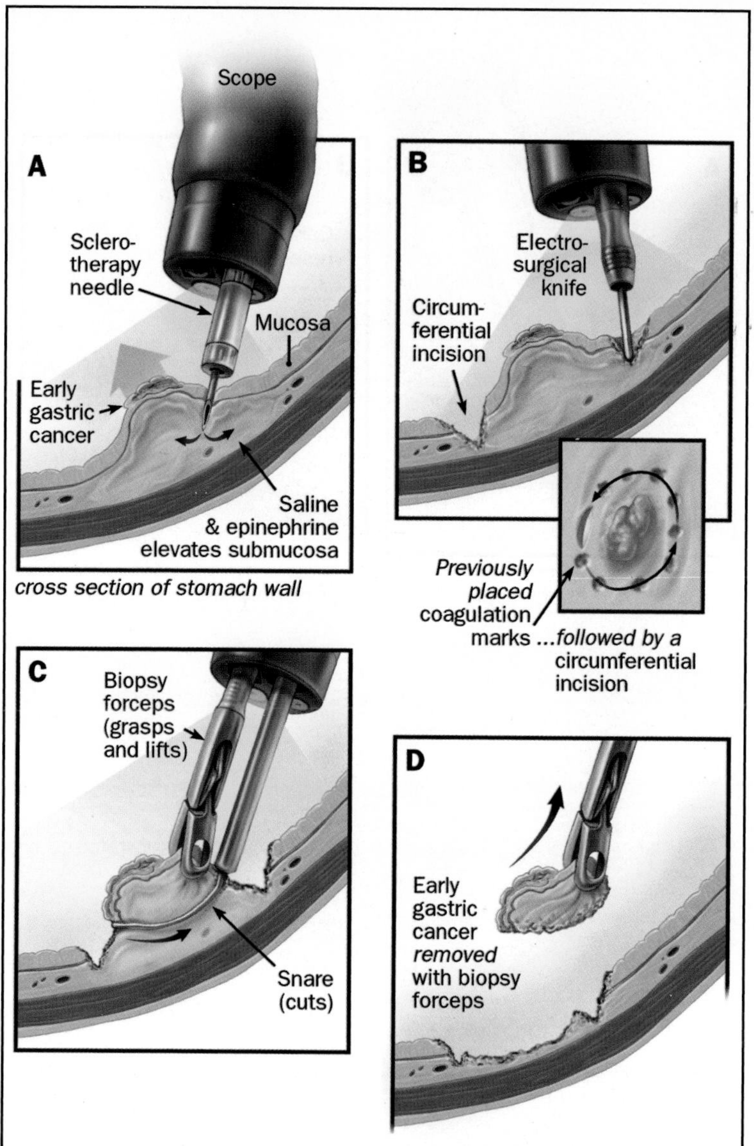

Figure 5-42. Endoscopic technique of strip biopsy.

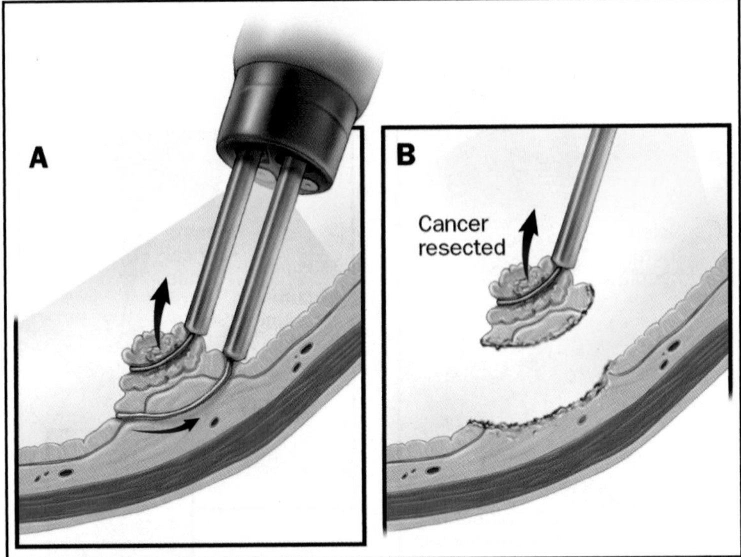

Figure 5-43. Endoscopic technique of double-snare polypectomy.

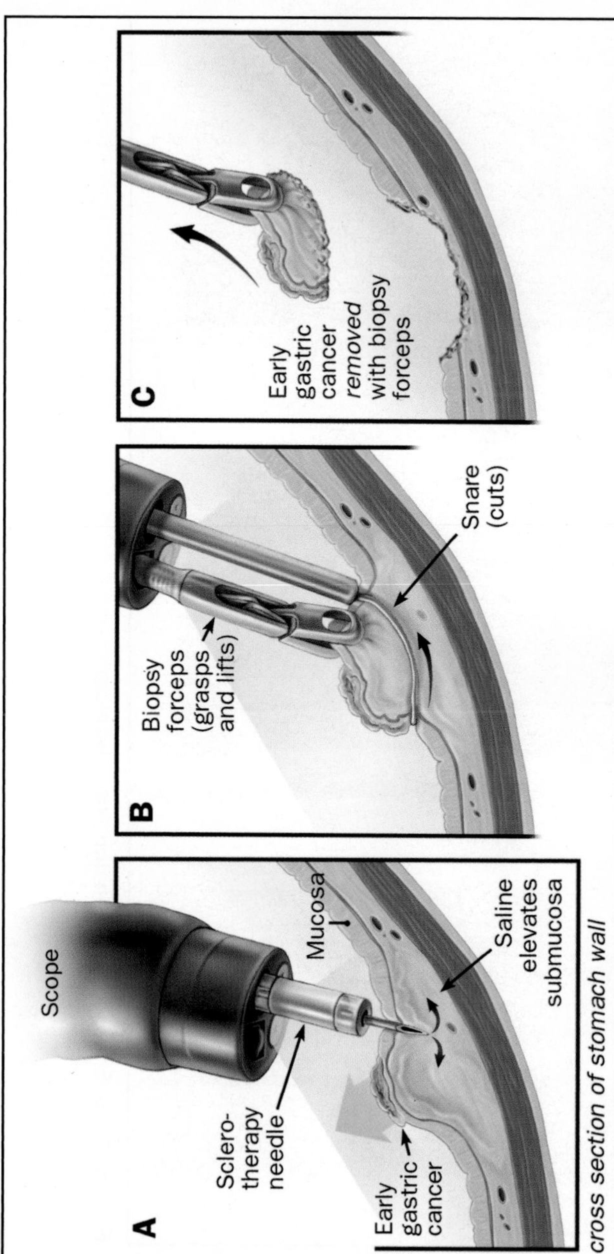

Figure 5-44. Endoscopic technique of saline and epinephrine.

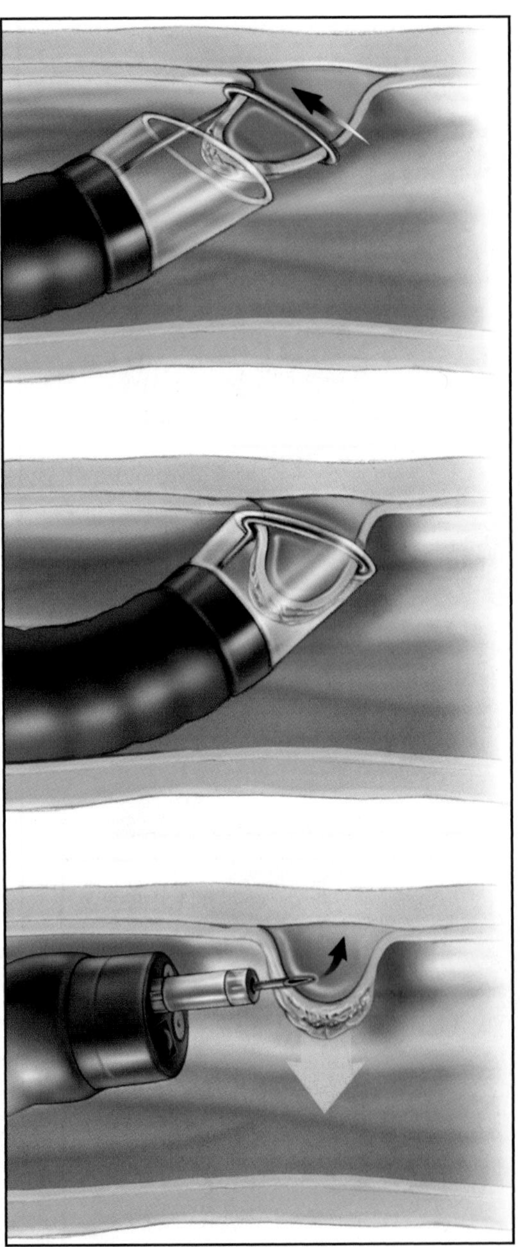

Figure 5-45. Endoscopic technique with clear-cap resection.

- ❖ Duette Multi-Band Mucosectomy is a system that uses a combined multi-band ligator device and snare which allows simple ligation and snare resection of superficial lesions and early lesions and early cancers in the upper GI tract (Figure 5-46).

Equipment

1. Same as for a diagnostic EGD.
2. Double-channel therapeutic upper endoscope
3. Sclerotherapy needle
4. Washing catheter
5. Two snares, one with electrocautery
6. Grasping forceps
7. Needle knife with cautery
8. Distal cap attachment
9. Cook Medical Duette Kit

Nursing Implications

Preprocedure

- ❖ Same as for a diagnostic EGD.
- ❖ Prophylactic antibiotics may be given at this time if appropriate.
- ❖ The administration of acid-reducing medication is important to reduce postoperative hemorrhage.

Intraprocedure

- ❖ Patient positioning: Same as for a diagnostic EGD.
- ❖ Patient monitoring: Same as for a diagnostic EGD.
- ❖ Topical anesthetic: Same as for a diagnostic EGD.
- ❖ Additional comfort measures: Same as for a diagnostic EGD.
- ❖ During the procedure, the nurse assists in the injection of agents, such as epinephrine 1:10,000.
- ❖ If the patient complains of pain when the snare strangulates the lesion or if the nonlifting sign is present, endoscopic mucosal resection is contraindicated.

Postprocedure

- ❖ Same as for a diagnostic EGD.
- ❖ The patient should be advised to adhere to a soft diet for 24 hours after EMR to prevent mechanical abrasion to the excised area.

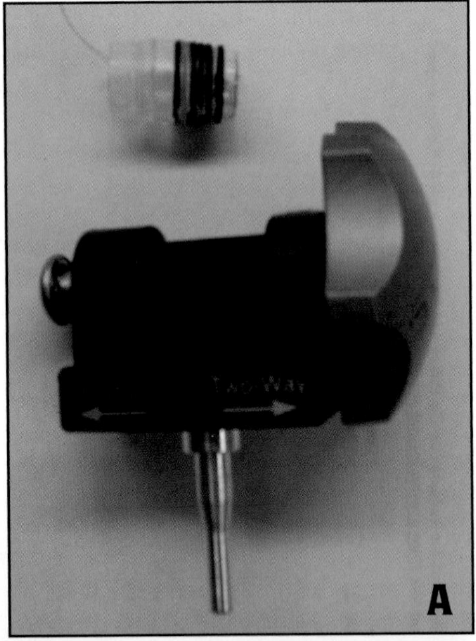

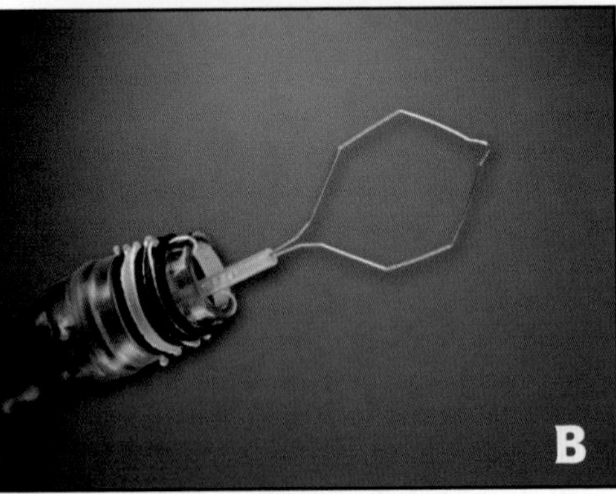

Figure 5-46. Duette handle (A) and snare (B).

- ❖ The patient should be instructed to avoid any medications that may increase the risk of bleeding (eg, aspirin) for 1 week after the procedure on the direction of the physician.
- ❖ Vomiting, hypotension, abdominal pain, or distention should be reported immediately to the physician.

Enteroscopy

Enteroscopy refers to the endoscopic examination of the small bowel. There are currently three types of small bowel enteroscopy.

The first type of enteroscopy is called double balloon push-pull enteroscopy. This technique involves the use of a balloon at the end of a special enteroscope camera and an overtube, which is a tube that fits over the endoscope, and is also fitted with a balloon. The procedure may be done with the use of moderate sedation or monitored anesthesia care. The enteroscope and overtube are inserted through the mouth and passed into the small bowel. Following this, the endoscope is advanced a small distance in front of the overtube and the balloon at the end is inflated. Using the assistance of friction at the point where the enteroscope and intestinal wall touch, the small bowel is accordioned back to the overtube. The overtube balloon is then deployed, and the enteroscope balloon is deflated. The process is then continued until the entire small bowel is inspected. The double-balloon enteroscope can also be passed in retrograde fashion, through the colon and into the ileum to inspect the end of the small bowel.

A second type of balloon enteroscopy has been developed using a single balloon. This balloon is positioned at the distal end of a plastic overtube that is placed over the insertion tube of a shorter enteroscope. The physician or the nurse may inflate or deflate the balloon with a foot pedal or hand control as the physician directs.

The third type of small bowel enteroscopy is called spiral enteroscopy. This is accomplished with a 55 F 130 cm overtube with a 5 mm raised element at the distal end. This overtube connects to a pediatric colonoscope and rotates independently so the doctor's visual perspective is not lost. Pleating of the small bowel is achieved by advancing the spiral segment of the overtube past the ligament of Treitz using the spiral technique. By disengaging the lock, the endoscope can be advanced in the traditional manner. To maximize insertion, two operators are required for doing spiral enteroscopy, one for the spiraling and one for the steering and insufflation.

Indications for enteroscopy are: iron deficiency anemia with normal colonoscopy and gastroscopy, bleeding from the GI tract of unknown origin, arterio-venous malformations, and ERCP in post-surgical patients with long afferent limbs.

EQUIPMENT

1. Video enterososcope or pediatric colonoscope (Figure 5-48)
2. Light source
3. 60 cc syringe with water for lubrication

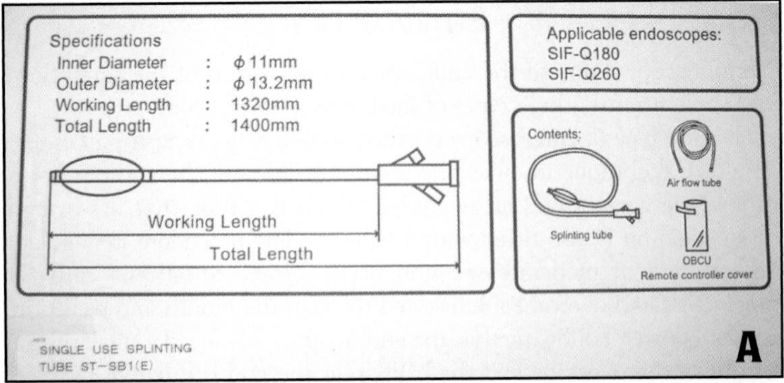

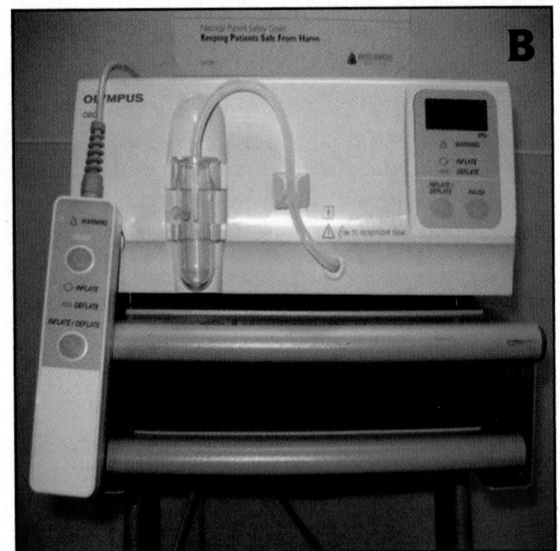

Figure 5-47. (A) Single balloon dimensions (diagram). (B) Balloon pump for single and double balloon enteroscope.

4. Bite block
5. Plastic overtubes with either single, double balloons or overtube with raised helical element at distal end
6. Fluoroscopy
7. Biopsy forceps

Nursing Implications

Preprocedure

- The patient should have nothing by mouth for 8 hours prior to the procedure.

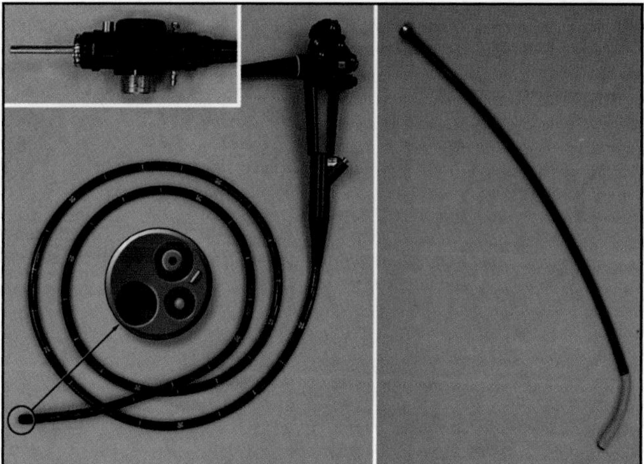

Figure 5-48. Push enteroscope with stiffening tube.

- ❖ Document baseline vital signs, blood pressure, pulse, respiration, oxygen saturation, level of consciousness, and pain level.
- ❖ Document medication allergies and daily medications, including dose and frequency.
- ❖ The physician should document a history and physical exam.
- ❖ The physician should obtain an informed consent from the patient or responsible adult.
- ❖ An intravenous infusion of D5/.45 normal saline (NS) should be started.
- ❖ Review discharge and follow-up instructions, including diet, activity, and possible untoward reactions, with the patient (or responsible adult) prior to sedation.
- ❖ Secure a responsible adult to accompany the patient home.

Intraprocedure

- ❖ Patient positioning: Left lateral position to facilitate drainage of secretions.
- ❖ Patient monitoring:
  1. Electrocardiogram, blood pressure, and pulse oximetry should be monitored every 2 minutes during administration of sedation and then documented every 5 minutes during the procedure.
  2. Emergency equipment including suction, oxygen, and crash cart must be readily available.
- ❖ Topical anesthetic: Viscous lidocaine "swish and swallow" or 4% lidocaine spray may be used.

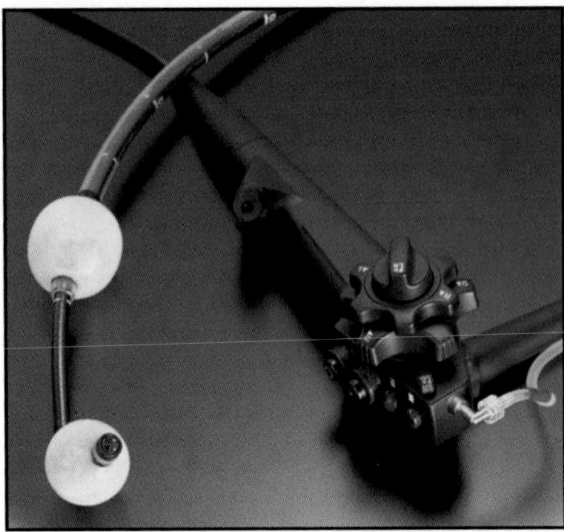

Figure 5-49A. Double balloon sheath and endoscope

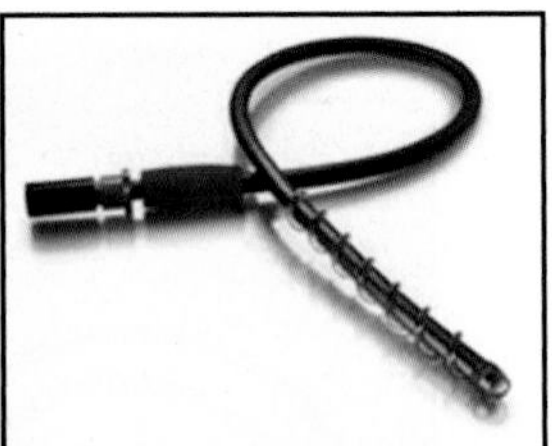

Figure 5-49B. Endo-ease for spiral endoscopy.

- Additional comfort measures:
  1. Place a pillow behind the patient's back for extra support while on his or her side.
  2. Soothing, calming words of encouragement along with light back massage may improve the patient's comfort.
- After the overtube is loaded onto the scope, lubricate the inside of the overtube with water using a 60 cc syringe attached to the port on the overtube.
- Fluoroscopy may be used to visualize position of the endoscope.
- Frequent suctioning may be necessary to prevent aspiration.
- It may be necessary to reposition the patient or apply pressure to the upper and midabdomen to facilitate passage of the endoscope.
- The physician may direct the nurse to inflate and deflate the balloon as neccessary (Figure 5-49).

Postprocedure

- The patient should be kept on his or her side until fully awake and able to control secretions.
- Monitor vital signs, blood pressure, pulse, respirations, oxygen saturation, and level of consciousness every 15 minutes (or more often if necessary) until they have returned to baseline.
- The patient may be discharged to home, accompanied by an adult with discharge instructions (see Appendix 3).
- The physician should be notified if the patient experiences vomiting, abdominal pain, distention, or fever.

Enteric Stent Placement

An enteric stent is an expandable metal mesh tube or plastic silicone coated tube used in patients with obstructive tumors of the duodenum, jejunum, or colon. Enteric stent placement is usually a palliative measure. The expandable enteric stent is advanced over a guidewire through the biopsy channel of the endoscope. Fluoroscopy is usually required for the insertion of the expandable metal stent. Dilation of the obstructed area may be necessary before stent placement (Figure 5-50).

Equipment

1. Upper endoscope or colonoscope
2. Mouthpiece for upper endoscopy
3. Topical anesthetic
4. Savary-Gilliard dilators and guidewire (Savary-Guillard guidewire or other .038-inch diameter guidewire) for the duodenal placement and balloon dilators with inflation device for colonic placement
5. Expandable metal enteral stents of assorted sizes (18 x 60 mm, 20 x 60 or 90 mm, and 22 x 60 or 90 mm)
6. Water-soluble lubricant
7. Fluoroscopy
8. Radiopaque markers and/or sclerotherapy needles with water-soluble contrast

Nursing Implications

Preprocedure

- Same as for diagnostic EGD or diagnostic colonoscopy.
- Prophylactic antibiotics may be given at this time if appropriate.
- The availability of stent sizes should be ascertained as soon as the procedure is scheduled. Stents are relatively expensive and may not be routinely stocked on the unit.

Intraprocedure

- Same as for diagnostic EGD or diagnostic colonoscopy.
- Patient positioning:
  1. The patient should be positioned in the left lateral or supine position on the fluoroscopy table.
  2. In order for the physician to approximate where the stent should be placed, radiopaque markers may be placed on the

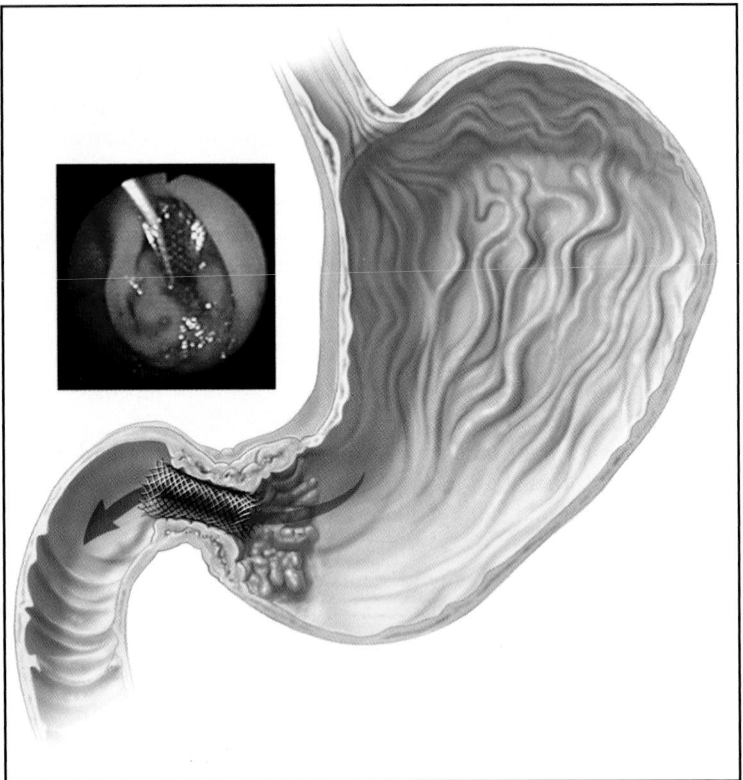

Figure 5-50. Location of an enteral stent in a patient with pyloric obstruction.

patient to be used as landmarks for stent placement, or alternatively, contrast may be injected into the upper and lower borders of the tumor.

3. The patient should be turned supine when using the fluoroscope to assess stent position.

- Patient monitoring: Same as for a diagnostic EGD.
- Additional comfort measures: Same as for a diagnostic EGD.

Postprocedure

- Same as for a diagnostic EGD.

Diagnostic Colonoscopy

Colonoscopy refers to the endoscopic examination of the large intestine (anus; rectum; sigmoid; descending, transverse, ascending colon; and rectum) (Figure 5-51).

Equipment

1. Colonoscope
2. Endoscopic light source
3. Water bottle
4. Colonic biopsy forceps
5. Bottles of formalin
6. Labels with patient's name
7. Suction apparatus

Additional Equipment That May be Needed

1. Cytology brushes
2. Requisition forms and labeled containers for cytopathology
3. Viral and fungal tubes for culture
4. Mucus traps

Nursing Implications

Preprocedure

Bowel, Diet, and Drug Modifications

- ❖ Prior to the procedure, the patient must undergo bowel cleansing:
  1. Colonic lavage (GoLYTELY [Braintree Laboratories, Braintree, Mass] or Colyte [Schwarz Pharma, Milwaukee, Wis]) requires a shorter amount of patient preparation time (approximately 4 to 6 hours) but may not be well-tolerated.
  2. Fleet phosphosoda kit (CB Fleet Co, Lynchburg, Va) requires a longer preparation time but may be better tolerated in some patients (should not be used in patients with impaired renal or cardiac function or the elderly)
  3. Cleansing tap water enemas are an alternative requiring a clear liquid diet for 2 days for patients who cannot tolerate the oral method.
  4. The nurse should be sure the patient has written instructions on the use of the bowel cleansing technique. If it is not pos-

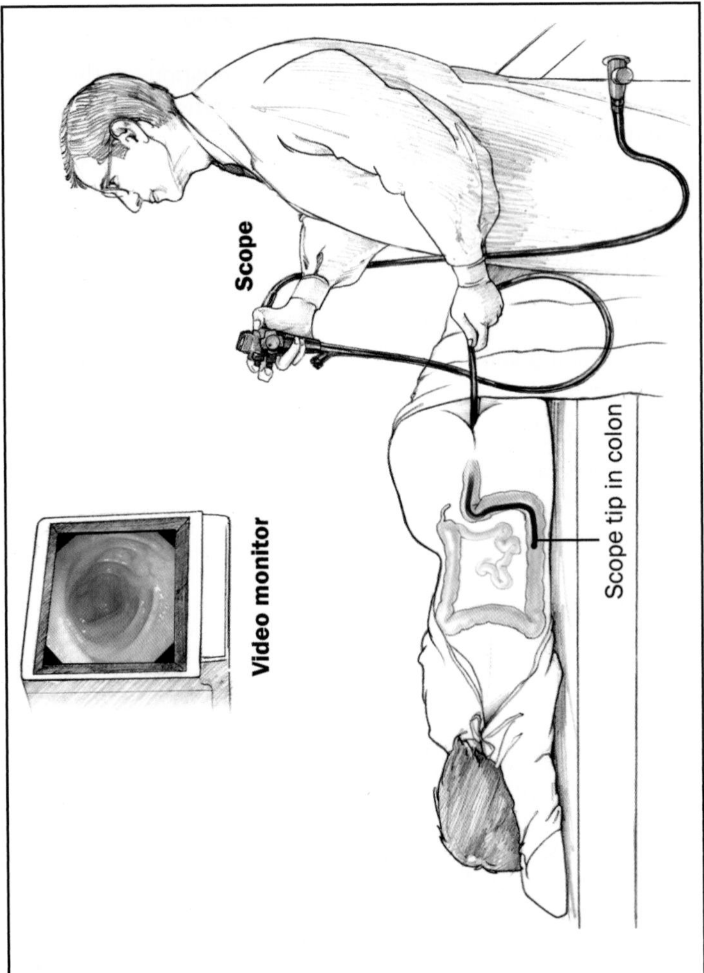

Figure 5-51. Patient positioning for colonoscopy.

sible to get written instructions to the patient in advance, a phone call with explicit instructions should be made several days prior to the test.

- The patient should refrain from using iron supplements (which may cause black staining of the bowel wall), aspirin, and NSAIDs 1 week prior to the procedure.

- ❖ Beets and red Jell-O should be avoided 24 to 48 hours prior to colonoscopy, as they may cause a reddish hue to the bowel contents.
- ❖ Anticoagulant therapy such as Coumadin (Bristol Myers Squibb, New York, NY) or heparin should be discontinued prior to the procedure on the advice of the physician. Generally, Coumadin is discontinued 1 week before the procedure and heparin may be discontinued 4 hours before the procedure.
- ❖ Secure a responsible adult to accompany the patient home.

Endoscopy Unit

- ❖ Document baseline blood pressure, pulse, respirations, oxygen saturation, and pain level.
- ❖ Document medication allergies and daily medications with dose and frequency.
- ❖ The physician should obtain an informed consent from the patient or responsible adult.
- ❖ Intravenous solution of D5/.45 NS or normal saline should be started.
- ❖ Discharge instructions should be read and signed by the patient or a responsible adult before sedation.

Intraprocedure

- ❖ Patient positioning: The left lateral position with the knees bent toward the chest facilitates insertion of the endoscope and fosters the comfort and privacy of the patient. The patient may be rotated during the procedure to facilitate passage of the endoscope.
- ❖ Patient monitoring:
  1. EKG, blood pressure, and pulse oximetry should be monitored every 2 minutes while administering the initial dose of sedation and then documented every 15 minutes during the procedure unless the patient's condition warrants more frequent monitoring.
  2. Vasovagal stimulation from excess air retention may cause belching and vomiting, therefore suction should be readily available.
  3. Oxygen via nasal cannula at 2 L may be administered when using IV moderate sedations.

- Nursing measures to facilitate passage of the colonoscope:
  1. The colonoscope may become looped during the course of colonoscopy. In this instance, the physician may require assistance from the nurse to apply abdominal pressure. Depending upon the area where the loop occurs, the physician will ask the nurse to exert flat pressure by using the palms of the hands. The loop often forms in the sigmoid colon, and by exerting flat pressure directly on the left lower quadrant, the endoscope may be advanced. This maneuver may be required at other points along the abdominal wall to facilitate endoscope passage.
  2. It is important not to apply excessive pressure to the patient's abdomen, as this may cause discomfort.
  3. If the physician is having difficulty advancing the endoscope to the cecum, it may be necessary to assist the patient in turning to a more supine, right side-down, or prone position.
  4. All specimens should be labeled, bagged, and sent to the laboratory. Virology cultures should be sent to the laboratory within 1 hour of collection.
- Additional comfort measures:
  1. Place a pillow behind the patient's back and between the knees to lend additional support and reduce pressure on the knees.
  2. Monitor vital signs for changes in pulse rate and blood pressure or expressions of verbal or nonverbal pain to keep the patient comfortable with intravenous medication.
  3. Soothing, calming words of encouragement along with light back massage may lessen the need for additional intravenous sedation.
  4. Try to maintain patient comfort and dignity at all times.
  5. The abdomen should be inspected and palpated frequently for distention; this may be alleviated by frequent suctioning via the endoscope.

Postprocedure

- The patient should be kept on his or her side until fully awake and able to control secretions.
- Vital signs, blood pressure, pulse, oxygen saturation, level of consciousness, and pain level should be monitored and documented every 15 minutes until they return to baseline, unless the patient's condition warrants more frequent monitoring.

- Approaches for the patient having difficulty expelling excess gas:
  1. Heat packs may be applied to the abdomen.
  2. The patient may be encouraged to change position frequently or tilt the pelvis by placing a pillow under the pelvis.
  3. Patients who are awake with stable vital signs may sit upright or be encouraged to ambulate.
  4. The nurse may insert a rectal tube just inside the anal canal to facilitate passage of colonic gas.
- The patient may be discharged home accompanied by an adult with discharge instructions (see Appendix 3).
- The physician should be notified if the patient experiences abdominal pain, pain radiating to the left shoulder tip (Kehr's sign), bleeding from the rectum, or has significant changes in vital signs.
- The patient should be advised to avoid the use of aspirin or NSAIDs for several days after polyp removal, as directed by the physician.

Chapter 5

Colonoscopy for Hemostasis

Colonoscopy for hemostasis may be performed to treat bleeding colon lesions such as bleeding neoplasms, arteriovenous malformations (AVMs), or other causes of bleeding in the colon.

Equipment

1. Same as for a diagnostic colonoscopy
2. Bipolar probe with energy unit
3. Epinephrine 1:10,000 and saline for injection
4. Sclerotherapy needle
5. Clipping device
6. Laser, APC, or cryotherapy unit

Nursing Implications

Preprocedure

Bowel, Diet, and Drug Modifications

- ❖ Same as for a diagnostic colonoscopy, except in situations of emergent bleeding.
- ❖ Purge lavage (may require nasogastric tube).

Endoscopy Unit

- ❖ Same as for a diagnostic colonoscopy.

Intraprocedure

- ❖ Patient positioning: Same as for a diagnostic colonoscopy.
- ❖ Patient monitoring: Same as for a diagnostic colonoscopy.
- ❖ Nursing measures to facilitate passage of the colonoscope: Same as for a diagnostic colonoscopy.
- ❖ Additional comfort measures: Same as for a diagnostic colonoscopy.

Postprocedure

- ❖ Same as for a diagnostic colonoscopy.

Colonoscopy With Polypectomy

Colonoscopy with polypectomy refers to the endoscopic removal of a colonic polyp using a snare with cautery, cold or hot biopsy forceps, or laser therapy (Figure 5-52).

Equipment

1. Same as for a diagnostic colonoscopy.
2. Biopsy forceps
3. Electrosurgical cautery unit or argon plasma coagulator
4. Polypectomy snare, grounding pad, and energy unit
5. Clipping device
6. Looping device
7. Laser
8. Sclerotherapy needle and epinephrine 1:10,000 or saline
9. Specimen trap
10. Tripod grasping forceps
11. Retrieval basket
12. Container with formalin labeled with the patient's name or other identifying information
13. Pathology requisition form

Nursing Implications

Preprocedure

Bowel, Diet, and Drug Modifications

- ❖ Same as for a diagnostic colonoscopy.

Endoscopy Unit

- ❖ Same as for a diagnostic colonoscopy.
- ❖ Prophylactic antibiotics may be given at this time if appropriate.

Intraprocedure

- ❖ Patient positioning: Same as for a diagnostic colonoscopy.
- ❖ Patient monitoring: Same as for a diagnostic colonoscopy.
- ❖ Nursing measures to facilitate passage of the colonoscope: Same as for a diagnostic colonoscopy.
- ❖ Additional comfort measures:
  1. Same as for a diagnostic colonoscopy.
  2. Reinforce that the removal of the polyp will be painless.

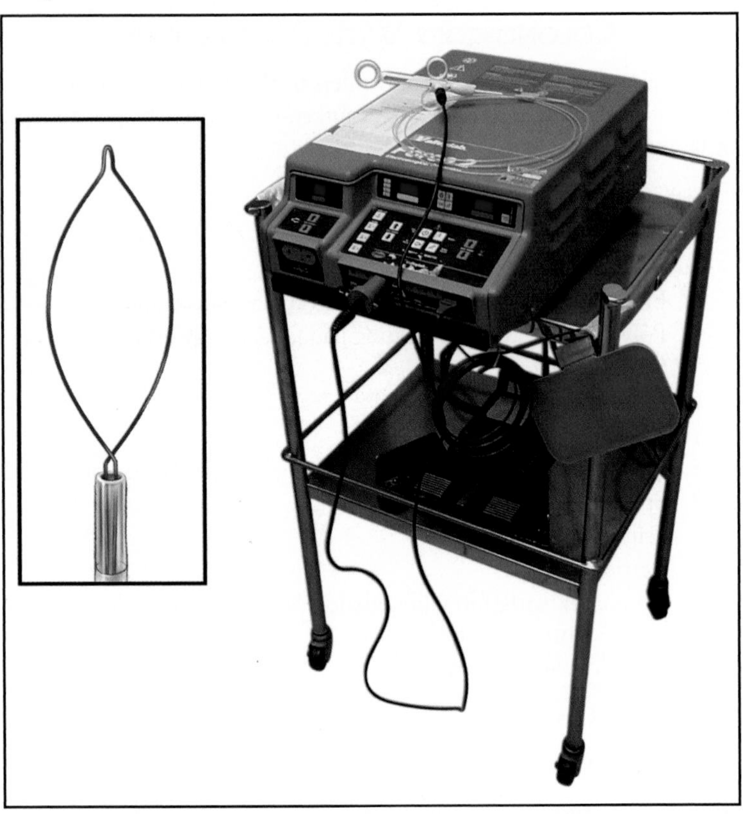

Figure 5-52. Electrosurgical unit with polypectomy snare and grounding pad.

- ❖ The patient should be grounded when using monopolar cautery for polyp removal (on the top portion of the thigh or the fleshy portion of the buttocks).

Postprocedure

- ❖ Same as for a diagnostic colonoscopy.
- ❖ The patient should be advised to avoid the use of aspirin or NSAIDs for several days after polyp removal, as directed by the physician.

COLONOSCOPY WITH DILATION

Dilations of the colon are performed for strictures from surgery, obstructing tumors, and inflammatory bowel disease. Through-the-scope (TTS) balloons are most often used for these types of dilations. A colonoscopy is performed to the point of the stricture. At this point, a lubricated balloon is passed through the biopsy channel of the endoscope and advanced to the midpoint of the structure. Fluoroscopy may be used to assist. The physician should direct the nurse to inflate the balloon while monitoring inflation pressure. The balloon is usually inflated for 1 minute. If necessary, the balloon may be reinflated several times. The physician may start with a small balloon and use increasingly larger balloons until the opening is large enough for passage of the endoscope.

EQUIPMENT

1. Same as for a diagnostic colonoscopy.
2. TTS colonic or anastomotic balloon dilators (see Figure 5-8C)
3. Inflation syringe gauge assembly
4. Sterile water to fill balloon (approximately 30 cc's)
5. Lubricant for balloon (vegetable oil spray)
6. Fluoroscopy

NURSING IMPLICATIONS

Preprocedure

Bowel, Diet, and Drug Modifications

- Same as for a diagnostic colonoscopy.

Endoscopy Unit

- Same as for a diagnostic colonoscopy.

Intraprocedure

- Patient positioning: Same as for a diagnostic colonoscopy.
- Patient monitoring: Same as for a diagnostic colonoscopy.
- Nursing measures to facilitate passage of the colonoscope: Same as for a diagnostic colonoscopy.
- Before handing the balloon dilator to the physician, the nurse should make sure it is well-lubricated with vegetable spray to facilitate passage through the biopsy channel of the colonoscope.

- Additional comfort measures: Same as for a diagnostic colonoscopy.

Postprocedure

- Same as for a diagnostic colonoscopy.

Diagnostic Sigmoidoscopy

Diagnostic sigmoidoscopy is the endoscopic examination of the anus, rectum, sigmoid, and descending colon. It is used to evaluate chronic diarrhea, fecal incontinence, ischemic colitis, lower gastrointestinal hemorrhage; to differentiate between bacterial dysentery, ulcerative colitis, and Crohn's disease; and as an adjunct to colorectal cancer screening.

Equipment

1. Video or fiberoptic flexible sigmoidoscope (Figure 5-53)
2. Light source
3. Water-soluble lubricant
4. Biopsy forceps
5. Formalin bottles and labels
6. Specimen trap
7. Viral culture tubes
8. Water bottle

Nursing Implications

Preprocedure

Bowel, Diet, and Drug Modifications

- ❖ Bowel cleansing:
  1. Magnesium citrate should be taken at 4 pm the day prior to the test, followed by a clear liquid supper.
  2. The patient should remain on clear liquids until after the test.
- ❖ One to 2 hours prior to the test, the patient should self-administer two Fleet enemas (or tap water enemas). Patients with diarrhea should not take enemas but should remain on clear liquids.
- ❖ No sedation is given for this exam unless the patient requests it. If sedation is given, the protocol for intravenous moderate sedation should be followed.

Endoscopy Unit

- ❖ The nurse will administer Fleet or tap water enemas if the patient was unable to self-administer.
- ❖ Baseline vital signs should be obtained including blood pressure, pulse, oxygen saturation, respirations, and pain level.
- ❖ Informed consent should be obtained.

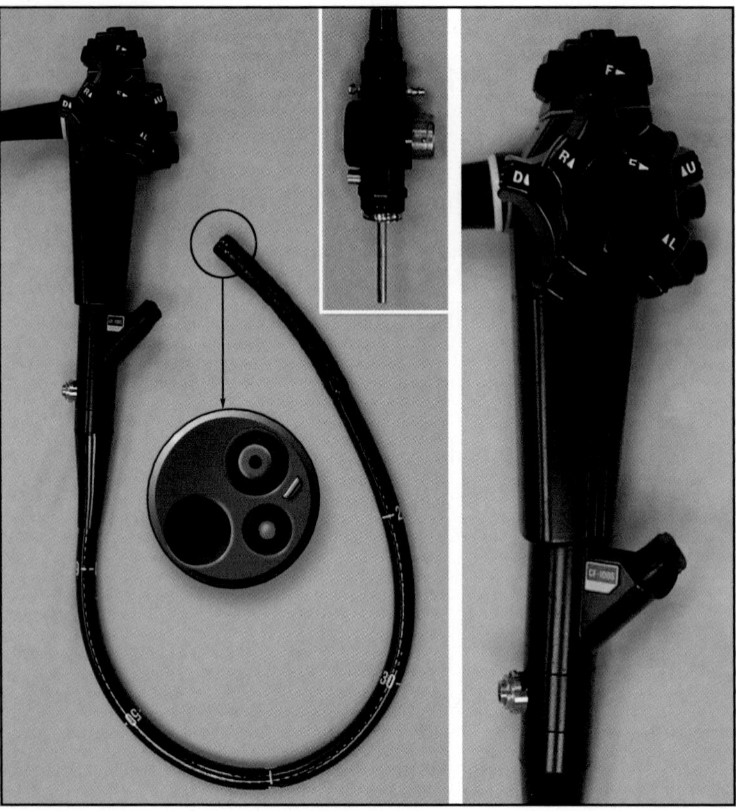

Figure 5-53. Flexible sigmoidoscope.

Intraprocedure

- Patient positioning:
  1. Patient is placed in the left lateral position with knees bent toward the chest.
  2. Keep the patient covered with minimal exposure.
- Patient monitoring (performed if sedation is used):
  1. EKG, blood pressure, and pulse oximetry should be monitored every 2 minutes while the initial dose of sedation is administered and then documented every 5 minutes unless the patient's condition warrants more frequent monitoring.

2. Suction should be readily available in case of vomiting from vasovagal stimulation or excess air retention.
3. Oxygen via nasal cannula at 2 L may be administered when using IV moderate sedation.

❖ Additional comfort measures:
1. Placing a pillow behind the patient's back and between the knees is helpful in keeping the patient on his or her side by lending support and reducing pressure between the knees.
2. Ongoing explanations of the procedure and visible images on the monitor may be helpful.
3. Soothing words of encouragement and light back massage may be helpful in providing emotional support.

Postprocedure

❖ All specimens should be labeled, bagged, and sent to the laboratory. Virology cultures should be sent to the laboratory within 1 hour of collection.

❖ Obtain vital signs including blood pressure, pulse, respirations, and pain level.

❖ If the patient did not receive sedation, he or she may be discharged with instructions (see Appendix 3) directly after the exam if vital signs are within normal limits and there are no signs of adverse reactions.

❖ If the patient was sedated, he or she should be kept on his or her side until fully awake and able to control secretions:
1. Monitor vital signs including blood pressure, pulse, respirations, oxygen saturation, pain level, and level of consciousness every 15 minutes (unless the patient's condition warrants more frequent monitoring) until they return to baseline.
2. The patient may be discharged home accompanied by an adult with discharge instructions (see Appendix 3).

❖ Patients undergoing screening flexible sigmoidoscopy receive instructions according to the findings of their exam.

Sigmoidoscopy with Infrared Coagulation

Infrared coagulation (IRC) is a non-surgical, non-invasive treatment for internal hemorroids. This treatment is quick and tolerated well by patients. No sedation is usually necessary. A small probe is inserted into the rectum through an anoscope. The sigmoidoscope is used to render light to the area being treated. The probe is attached to a unit that emits an infrared light hot enough to coagulate the hemorrhoid upon touch, causing it to eventually recede. The patient may experience heat, but not pain.

Equipment

1. Same as for diagnostic sigmoidoscopy.
2. IRC unit and probe (Figure 5-54)
3. Anoscope

Nursing Implications

Preprocedure

- Same as for diagnostic sigmoidoscopy.

Intraprocedure

- Same as for diagnostic sigmoidoscopy.

Post Procedure

- Same as for diagnostic colonoscopy, except:
  1. Patient should remain on a low fiber soft diet or full liquid diet for that day and that evening.
  2. Do not manipulate your rectum for 1 week (no enemas or suppositories).
  3. No strenuous exercise for 1 week (no biking, running or weight lifting).

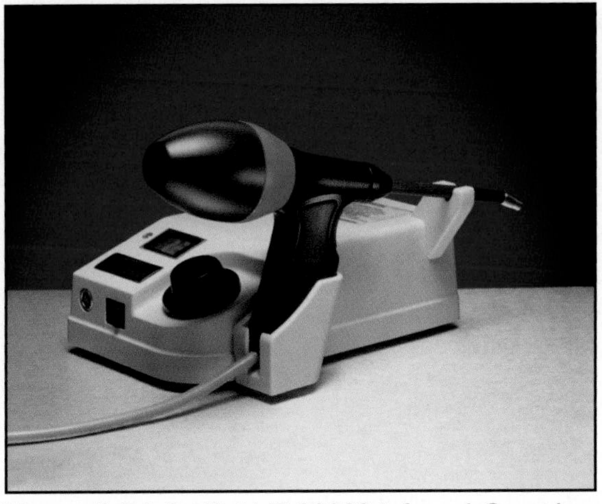

Figure 5-54. Redfield IRC2100 Infrared Coagulator.

Chapter 5

Anal Dilation With Hagar Dilators

Hagar dilators are incremental metal sounds that are used to gradually dilate strictures of the anal canal (after ileoanal pull-through or other surgical or functional stricture of the anus). This may be done in conjunction with flexible sigmoidoscopy or by itself after digital rectal exam.

Equipment

1. Hagar incremental dilators (Figure 5-55)
2. Water-soluble lubricant
3. Flexible sigmoidoscope

Nursing Implications

Preprocedure

Bowel, Diet, and Drug Modifications

- No bowel preparation is necessary unless the physician is going to perform flexible sigmoidoscopy. If this is the case, preparation is the same as for diagnostic sigmoidoscopy.
- If sedation is not used, the patient may have a clear liquid supper at 4 pm. At 6 pm the patient should take one bottle of magnesium citrate followed by two 8-oz glasses of water.
- The day of the procedure, two Fleet enemas may be self-administered 1 hour before arriving at the endoscopy unit.
- Patients unable to self-administer the Fleet enemas should arrive at the endoscopy unit at least 2 hours earlier so the nurse can administer them.
- The nurse should call the patient a day or two prior to the procedure to clarify the instructions and make adjustments as needed.

Endoscopy Unit

- If sedation is to be used, follow the same protocol for sedation as for diagnostic colonoscopy.
- Prophylactic antibiotics may be administered at this time if appropriate.
- If sedation is not used, baseline vital signs are taken before the procedure.

Intraprocedure

- Patient positioning: Same as for a diagnostic colonoscopy.

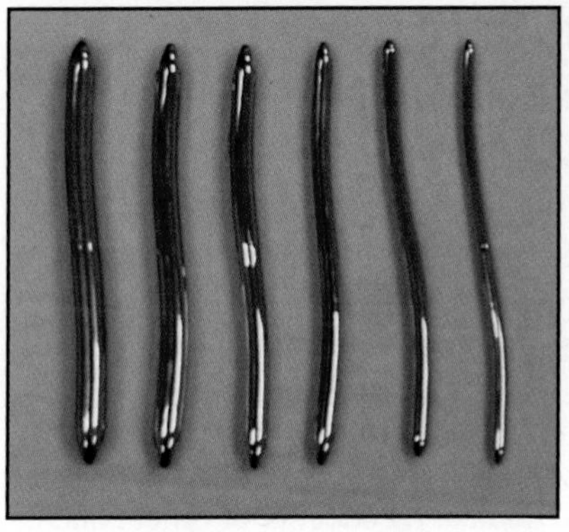

Figure 5-55. Hagar dilators.

- Patient monitoring:
  1. If sedation is used, monitoring is the same as for diagnostic colonoscopy.
  2. If sedation is not used, no intraprocedure monitoring is necessary.
- Additional comfort measures:
  1. If sedation is not used, the nurse will need to provide emotional support with calm, soothing words of encouragement and light back massage.
  2. It is a good idea to have dilators and lubricant warmed (in a pan of warm water) before use.

Postprocedure

- If sedation is used, the procedure is the same as for a diagnostic colonoscopy.
- If sedation is not used:
  1. Vital signs should be obtained at the end of the procedure.
  2. The patient may be discharged as long as there are no untoward reactions, bleeding, or perforation.
- Warm-water baths may be recommended for patient comfort.
- The patient should be advised of the signs of infection and to watch for symptoms.
- Stool softeners may be beneficial to make bowel movements less painful.
- Patients should be advised to eat a high-fiber diet.

Chapter 5

Endoscopic Retrograde Cholangiopancreatography

Endoscopic retrograde cholangiopancreatography (ERCP) is an endoscopic procedure in which the biliary and pancreatic ductal systems are visualized under fluoroscopy by injection of radiopaque contrast. ERCP is used to diagnose and treat disorders of the biliary system (eg, obstructive jaundice, disease of the intra- or extrahepatic biliary system, pancreatic cancer, and recurrent pancreatitis of unknown etiology). ERCP is also used to assess pancreatic and ductal anatomy prior to operative, radiologic, or endoscopic intervention for chronic pancreatitis, suspected pancreatic trauma, pseudocyst, or other pancreaticobiliary disorders.

Equipment

1. Side-viewing endoscope (duodenoscope) (Figure 5-56)
2. Bite block
3. Light source
4. Water bottle
5. Wall suction, liner, and suction tubing with mouth suction
6. Emesis basin
7. Gauze 4x4 pads
8. Water-soluble lubricant
9. Ionic contrast agent and 20-cc syringes
10. ERCP catheters of various types (tapered, ultratapered, ball tip, cone tip, needle tip, and standard tip; check for physician preference prior to each case) (Figure 5-57)
11. Electrical grounding pad for possible sphincterotomy
12. Lead aprons and thyroid shields
13. Fluoroscopy

ERCP

Additional Equipment That May be Needed

1. Biopsy forceps long enough to fit through a duodenoscope
2. Biliary cytology brushes
3. Specimen bottles with formalin
4. Washing catheters
5. 10-cc syringes for aspirating bile or pancreatic fluid

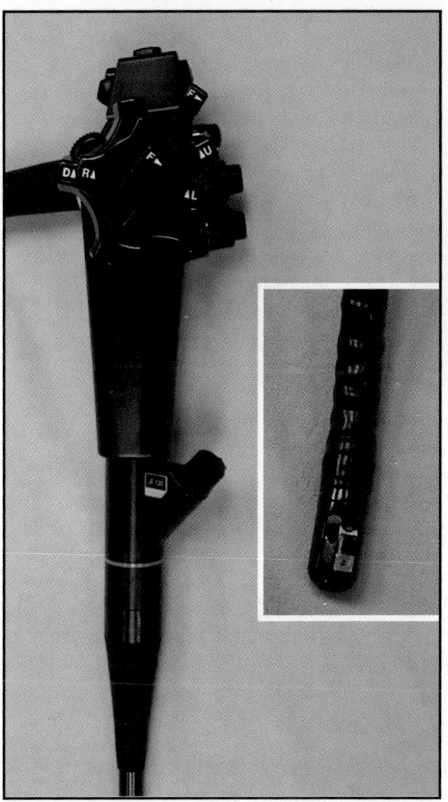

Figure 5-56. Duodenoscope.

Nursing Implications

Preprocedure

- ❖ The patient should have nothing by mouth for 8 hours prior to the procedure.
- ❖ Monitor baseline vital signs, including blood pressure, pulse, respirations, pain level, and oxygen saturation.
- ❖ Medication allergies and daily medications, including dose and frequency, should be documented.
- ❖ The physician should obtain an informed consent.
- ❖ An intravenous of D5/.45 NS or .9 NS should be in place.

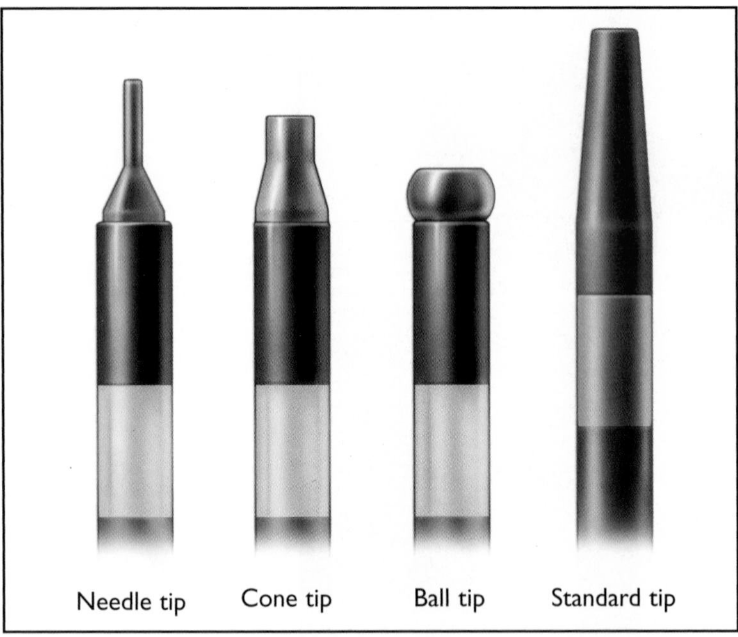

Figure 5-57. Types of ERCP diagnostic catheters.

- ❖ Prophylactic antibiotics should be given at this time if appropriate.
- ❖ The physician should be notified of ionic drug allergies. Depending upon the severity of the allergy, steroids or an antihistamine may be prescribed before the procedure. Nonionic dye should be used in this subgroup of patients.
- ❖ Discharge instructions should be read and signed by the patient or responsible adult before sedation (see Appendix 3).
- ❖ Secure a responsible adult to accompany the patient home.

Intraprocedure

- ❖ Patient positioning:
  1. The patient should be placed in the left lateral position with his or her left arm behind the back (this facilitates turning the patient into the prone position during the procedure).
  2. Secure proper body alignment to prevent nerve damage to extremities (this may require the use of an arm guard or body wedge).

- ❖ Patient monitoring:
  1. EKG, blood pressure, and pulse oximetry should be performed and documented every 2 minutes during the initial induction of sedation, then every 15 minutes unless the patient's condition warrants more frequent monitoring.
- ❖ Emergency equipment, including suction, oxygen, and crash cart, must be readily available.
- ❖ Topical anesthesia: Viscous lidocaine swish and swallow or 4% lidocaine spray may be used to facilitate insertion of the endoscope.
- ❖ Additional comfort measures:
  1. Frequent suctioning is important to keep the patient comfortable and the airway clear.
  2. A wedge may be placed under the patient's chest to provide support while he or she is positioned on his or her side.
  3. Patients may feel claustrophobic and uncomfortable; supportive nursing care is extremely important in consoling the patient and obtaining cooperation.
- ❖ Flush a standard ERCP catheter with dye before the procedure begins.
- ❖ It is important to keep the catheter free of air bubbles because they interfere with the diagnosis of stones. When looking for stones, it is best to use half-strength dye (50 cc of dye with 50 cc of sterile water) for easier visualization.
- ❖ When the physician has determined the placement of the catheter in the bile or pancreatic duct, he or she may ask the nurse to inject the dye:
  1. Gentle injection pressure should be used when infusing contrast to decrease the risk of pancreatitis.
  2. A 20-cc syringe is commonly used because smaller-size syringes generate greater forces.
  3. Patients who have been on narcotics for long periods of time are often resistant to sedation. If sufficient medication has been administered and the patient is still not comfortable, the procedure should be terminated and other forms of sedation used, such as propofol (an anesthetic agent). Propofol use is not considered moderate sedation and may not be administered by an RN (Figure 5-58).

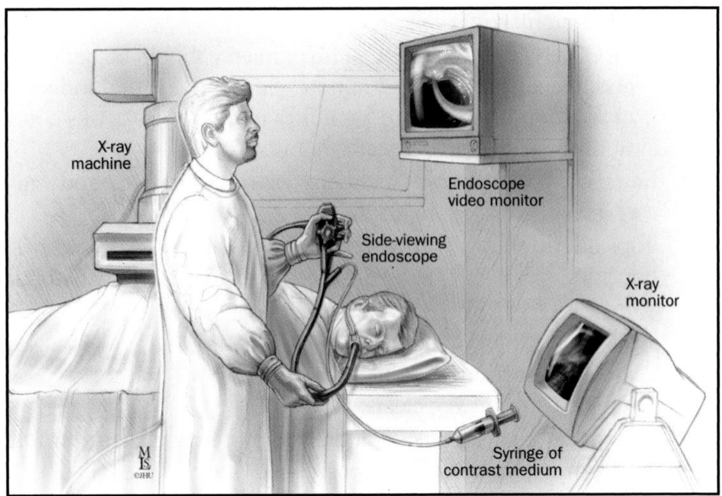

Figure 5-58. Patient set-up for ERCP.

Postprocedure

- ❖ Keep the patient on his or her side until fully awake and able to control secretions.
- ❖ Monitor vital signs, blood pressure, pulse, respirations, oxygen saturation, level of pain, and consciousness until the patient returns to baseline.
- ❖ Recovery after ERCP may be longer depending upon the amount of sedation used.
- ❖ Complications of ERCP include pancreatitis and perforation, which may be manifested by worsening abdominal pain, vomiting, fever, and chills. The physician should be notified if these complications are suspected.
- ❖ If the patient's recovery is uneventful, he or she may be released in the company of a responsible adult with discharge instructions (see Appendix 3).

Chapter 5

ERCP With Sphincterotomy

A sphincterotomy is an incision made into the sphincter of Oddi. The indications include common bile duct stone removal, endoscopic stent placement, and treatment of sphincter of Oddi dysfunction. A pancreatic sphincterotomy may also be performed in cases of biliary pancreatitis, pancreas divisum, and pancreatic stones.

An ERCP is performed to visualize the pancreatic or biliary ducts. The sphincterotomy is performed by inserting an endoscopic sphincterotome into the biopsy channel of a side-viewing duodenoscope. The sphincterotome is advanced into the papilla and strategically placed within the sphincter. During the procedure, the patient is grounded and the sphincterotome is connected to a cautery unit. The physician determines the cautery unit settings. Once the sphincterotomy is performed, the patient is ready for stone removal, stent placement, or dilation of the ducts.

Equipment

1. Duodenoscope (may need a therapeutic duodenoscope if a stent larger than 7 Fr is being placed)
2. Light source
3. Water bottle
4. Gauze 4x4 pads
5. Variety of ERCP catheters (standard, taper tip, ultrataper tip, cone tip, ball tip, needle tip)
6. Sphincterotome with activator cord (Figure 5-59)
7. Grounding pad
8. Electrosurgical cautery unit or argon plasma coagulator with foot pedal
9. Contrast medium and 20-cc syringes
10. Guidewires
11. 60-cc syringe with sterile water for flushing catheters and sphincterotomes

Additional Equipment That May be Needed

1. Epinephrine diluted to 1:10,000 if bleeding occurs
2. Various stone-removal balloons used for tamponade in the case of bleeding
3. Various extraction baskets

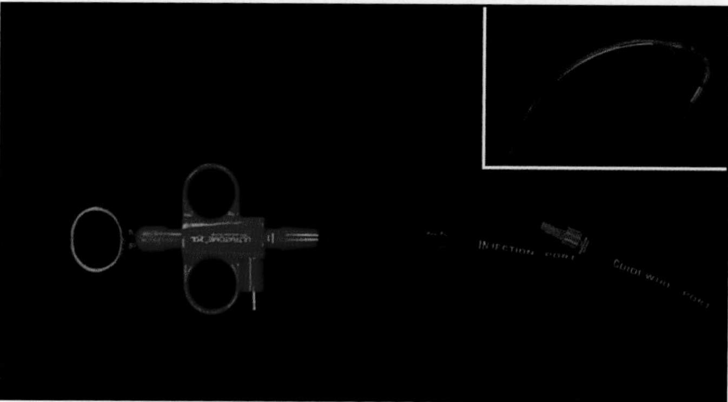

Figure 5-59. Sphincterotome.

Nursing Implications

Preprocedure

- ❖ Same as for ERCP.
- ❖ Medications containing aspirin, ibuprofen, or medications that alter the bleeding time (eg, anticoagulants) should be discontinued on the physicians' order for at least 1 week prior to the procedure.
- ❖ The physician may order an antibiotic to be given intravenously 1 hour before the procedure, if appropriate.
- ❖ The patient should have recent coagulation studies.
- ❖ It may be necessary to admit the patient after the procedure; pre-planning for admission may be necessary.

Intraprocedure

- ❖ Patient positioning: Same as for ERCP.
- ❖ Patient monitoring: Same as for ERCP.
- ❖ Topical anesthetic: Same as for ERCP.
- ❖ Additional comfort measures: Same as for ERCP.
- ❖ The patient must be grounded to prevent burns occurring during sphincterotomy. Most modern cautery units will not function unless the grounding pad is properly placed and attached.
- ❖ Flush the papillotome with 2 cc of contrast dye and/or load with a guidewire (physicians' preference).

- It is the nurse's or assistant's responsibility to assist the physician in the manipulation of the sphincterotome.
- Once dye is injected through the sphincterotome, flush the channel with sterile water before a guidewire or glidewire is used.
- If excessive bleeding occurs after sphincterotomy, the physician may request epinephrine diluted to 1:10,000 flushed through a sclerotherapy needle or injected around the bleeding site. Sometimes tamponade may be accomplished by using an inflated stone retrieval balloon pressed against the bleeding site.

Postprocedure

- Same as for ERCP.
- The physician should advise the patient about the resumption of anticoagulants.

ERCP With Stone Extraction

Biliary duct or pancreatic stone removal may be accomplished in a variety of ways. The physician may choose to use a basket, a stone-retrieval balloon, or a lithotriptor for removal.

The basket may be four-wire, eight-wire memory, or double lumen (contrast can be injected through one port and a guidewire can be inserted through another port). When using a basket, the ERCP is performed and the stones are located under fluoroscopy. A sphincterotomy may be performed to facilitate passage of the stone(s). A basket is inserted into the bile duct, advanced to a level above the stone(s), and opened. While pulling the basket through the duct it is usually closed and then removed with the stones inside. If stones are retrieved, the basket is reopened and the stones are released into the duodenum and passed in the stool. This procedure can be repeated several times until all stones are removed.

Another method of stone extraction utilizes a stone-retrieval balloon. ERCP is performed and the stones are located with fluoroscopy. The catheter is withdrawn and a stone extraction balloon is inserted into the bile duct through the biopsy channel of the endoscope. Typically, a sphincterotomy is performed before the insertion of the balloon. The balloon is then advanced to a level above the stone, inflated, and then used to extract the stone. The procedure may be repeated several times until the duct is clear of stones. The balloons are available in three sizes: 8.5 mm, 11.5 mm, and 15 mm; physician preference will determine the size(s) selected.

One method of stone removal is lithotripsy. After performance of the ERCP with stone visualization, the cannula is withdrawn and a biliary lithotriptor (a device with stone crushing capability) is used. A basket-type instrument is inserted into the bile duct. A wire running from the basket through the biopsy channel of the endoscope is brought externally to a winding device. The winding device contracts the basket tightly around the stones and crushes them. The stone-retrieval balloon is inserted into the duct, and the smaller crushed stones are swept into the duodenum. The lithotriptor is typically used when the stones are larger than 12 to 15 mm.

Equipment

❖ Same as for ERCP with sphincterotomy.

Additional Equipment That May be Needed

1. Stone retrieval baskets (Figure 5-60)
2. Stone retrieval balloons (Figure 5-61)
3. Biliary lithotriptor (Figure 5-62)

Nursing Implications

Preprocedure

- Same as for ERCP with sphincterotomy.

Intraprocedure

- Patient positioning: Same as for ERCP with sphincterotomy.
- Patient monitoring: Same as for ERCP with sphincterotomy.
- Topical anesthesia: Same as for ERCP with sphincterotomy.
- Additional comfort measures: Same as for ERCP with sphincterotomy.
- If excessive bleeding occurs after sphincterotomy, the physician may request epinephrine diluted to 1:10,000 or NS flushed through a sclerotherapy needle to be injected around the bleeding incision.
- Before the basket is put through the biopsy channel of the endoscope, the nurse should check to make sure the working parts are functioning properly. The physician may decide to load the basket with a wire or flush it with dye before insertion.
- The physician will direct the nurse to open the basket after it is advanced to a level above the stones. As the physician pulls the basket back, he or she will direct the nurse to close it.
- The sphincterotome is removed over the guidewire or glidewire and the balloon is inserted. When the exchange begins, the nurse's responsibility is to apply steady forward pressure to the guidewire as the physician is withdrawing the ERCP cannula. This keeps the guidewire in position within the duct. Communication between nurse and physician is essential for success.
- Intermittent fluoroscopy may be used to make sure the guidewire is in place (if marked guidewires are used, it lessens the need for fluoroscopy).
- The balloon should be checked for holes before it is inserted into the biopsy channel.

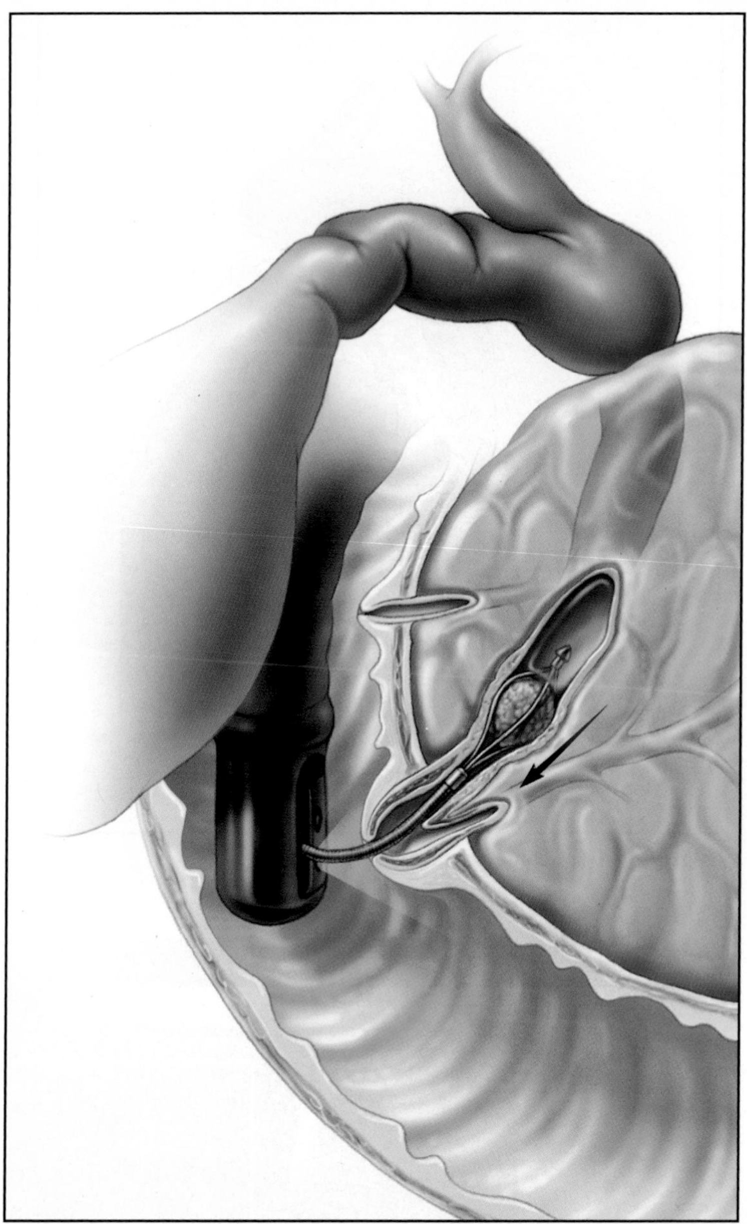

Figure 5-60. Stone retrieval basket.

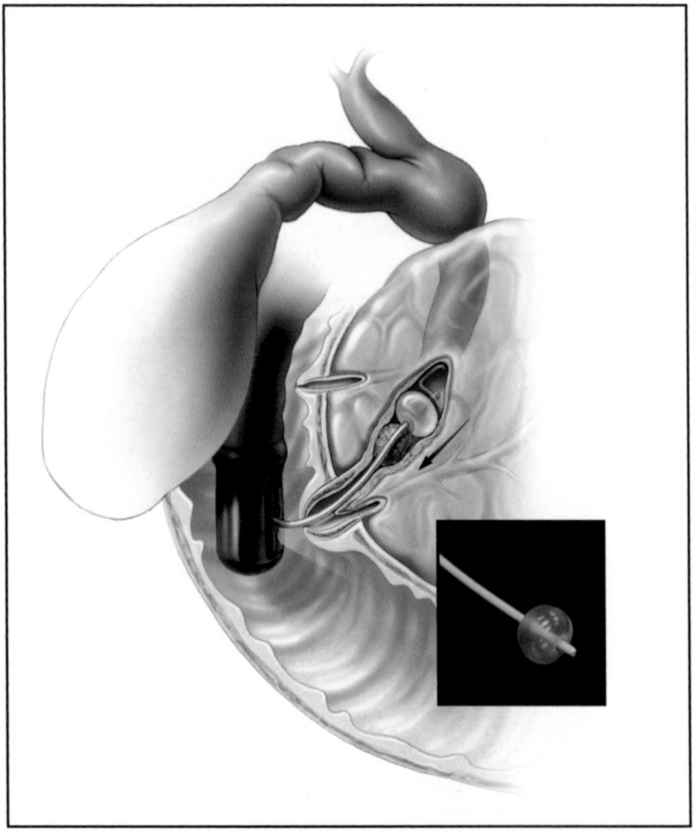

Figure 5-61. Stone retrieval balloon.

Figure 5-62. Endoscopic lithotriptor.

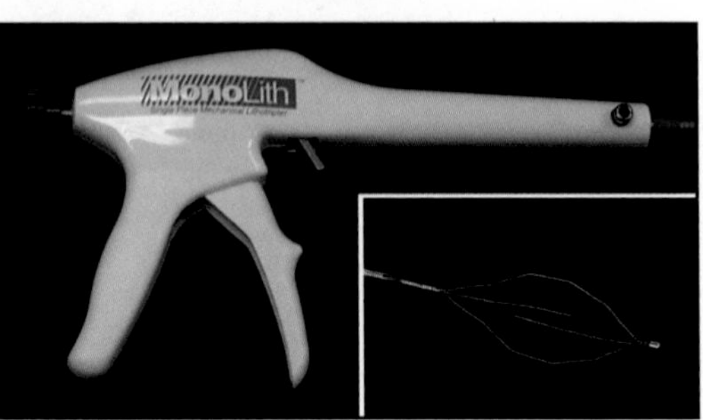

- ❖ The nurse will be instructed to inflate the balloon once it is positioned. The nurse should check the balloon specifications (on the packaging) for the proper amount of air inflation. The physician will direct the nurse to inflate or deflate the balloon as needed.
- ❖ The nurse should check with the physician in advance to see if the lithotriptor will be needed for stone crushing. It is the responsibility of the nurse to assemble it.

Postprocedure

- ❖ Same as for ERCP with sphincterotomy.

Chapter 5

ERCP WITH BILIARY DILATION

Biliary dilation is used to treat strictures caused by sclerosing cholangitis, bile duct injuries, or inoperable bile duct malignancies. Dilating balloons come in three sizes: 4 mm, 6 mm, and 8 mm in diameter. A sphincterotomy may be performed before the dilation (at the physicians' discretion). A guidewire is passed through the biopsy channel of a side-viewing duodenoscope and advanced to a point beyond the stricture. Once the balloon is placed across the stricture, a syringe filled with half-strength dye and a manometer is attached to the balloon port. The physician will direct the nurse to inflate the balloon to the desired pressure, usually for up to 1 minute. The procedure may be repeated several times until complete dilation of the duct is achieved.

EQUIPMENT

- ❖ Same as for ERCP with sphincterotomy.

Additional Equipment That May be Needed

1. Therapeutic endoscope may be required (if larger than a 7-Fr stent is being placed)
2. ERCP contrast dye and 20-cc syringes
3. Guidewires (physician's discretion)
4. Various sizes of biliary plastic and expandable stents (physician's discretion)

NURSING IMPLICATIONS

Preprocedure

- ❖ Same as for ERCP with sphincterotomy.

Intraprocedure

- ❖ Patient positioning: Same as for ERCP with sphincterotomy.
- ❖ Patient monitoring: Same as for ERCP with sphincterotomy.
- ❖ Topical anesthetic: Same as for ERCP with sphincterotomy.
- ❖ Additional comfort measures: Same as ERCP with sphincterotomy.
- ❖ It is important for the nurse to have different sizes of biliary balloons close at hand; balloon size is determined after the physician assesses the size of the stricture on x-ray.
- ❖ It is not necessary to inflate the balloons prior to use because once inflated, the low profile is lost, making it more difficult to

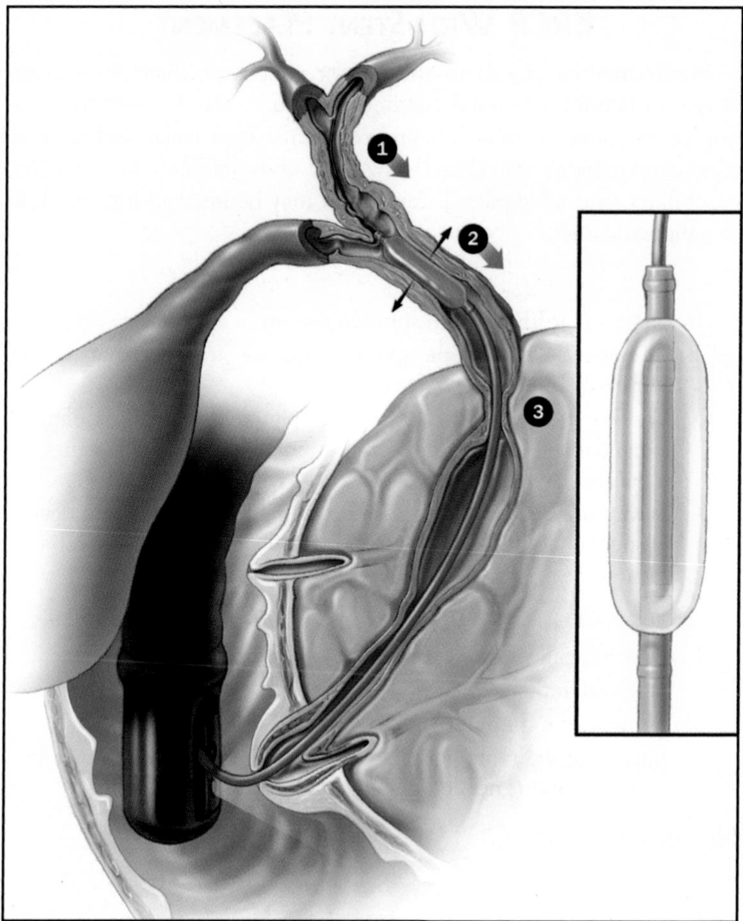

Figure 5-63. Endoscopic technique of stricture dilation with dilating balloon.

advance through strictures. The sphincterotome will be removed and the dilating balloon will be threaded over the guidewire and pushed into position (Figure 5-63).

Postprocedure

- Same as for ERCP with sphincterotomy.

Chapter 5

ERCP With Stent Placement

Stents may be placed in the bile or pancreatic duct, most commonly to maintain luminal patency. They may also be used for dilation of strictures, to treat bile and pancreatic duct leaks, and to treat pancreatic pseudocysts. There is a variety of stents, including straight, nasobiliary, or double pigtail stents, that may be inserted into the bile or pancreatic duct.

Equipment

1. Same as for ERCP with sphincterotomy.
2. Therapeutic endoscope may be required (if larger than a 7-Fr stent is being placed).
3. Various sizes of plastic biliary and pancreatic stents, including expandable biliary stents or nasobiliary and pigtail stents, as requested by physician.
4. Stents may be packaged as a kit and include stent, guidewire, pusher tubes, and catheters; additional stents may be purchased separately.

Additional Equipment That May be Needed

1. Dilating balloons or catheters
2. Sclerotherapy needle
3. Epinephrine diluted to 1:10,000 if bleeding occurs
4. Various stone removal balloons used for tamponading bleeding (see equipment needed for ERCP with sphincterotomy)

Nursing Implications

Preprocedure

- Same as for ERCP with sphincterotomy.

Intraprocedure

- Patient positioning: Same as for ERCP with sphincterotomy.
- Patient monitoring: Same as for ERCP with sphincterotomy.
- Topical anesthetic: Same as for ERCP with sphincterotomy.
- Additional comfort measures: Same as for ERCP with sphincterotomy.
- The physician will determine the size of the stent needed. If the stent being used is larger than 7 Fr, a larger channel or therapeutic side-viewing duodenoscope will be required.

- The nurse may be required to assist with wire exchanges during the procedure. The nurse will be responsible for maintaining the guidewire position by applying steady forward pressure on the guidewire as the physician is withdrawing the ERCP cannula. Intermittent fluoroscopy may be used to confirm guidewire placement. The need for fluoroscopy is decreased when using marked guidewires.
- Stents larger than 7 Fr in diameter require the use of a guiding catheter. After the stent is threaded over the guiding catheter, a pusher tube may be used to advance the stent through the biopsy channel of the endoscope. The physician may request that the nurse place continuous backward pressure on the guidewire and guiding catheter. This will assist the passage of the stent over the guiding catheter and into the duct.
- Nasobiliary stent placement is performed directly over the guidewire using a pusher tube to advance the stent. Once the stent has been positioned in the duct, it is externalized through the mouth and the endoscope is withdrawn. The nasobiliary tube is then rerouted through the nose for patient comfort. The tube must be securely taped to the patient's nose and neck (Figures 5-64 and 5-65).

Postprocedure

- Same as for ERCP with sphincterotomy.
- Drainage from the nasobiliary tube should be measured and documented. Any change in color, volume, or odor should be reported to the physician.

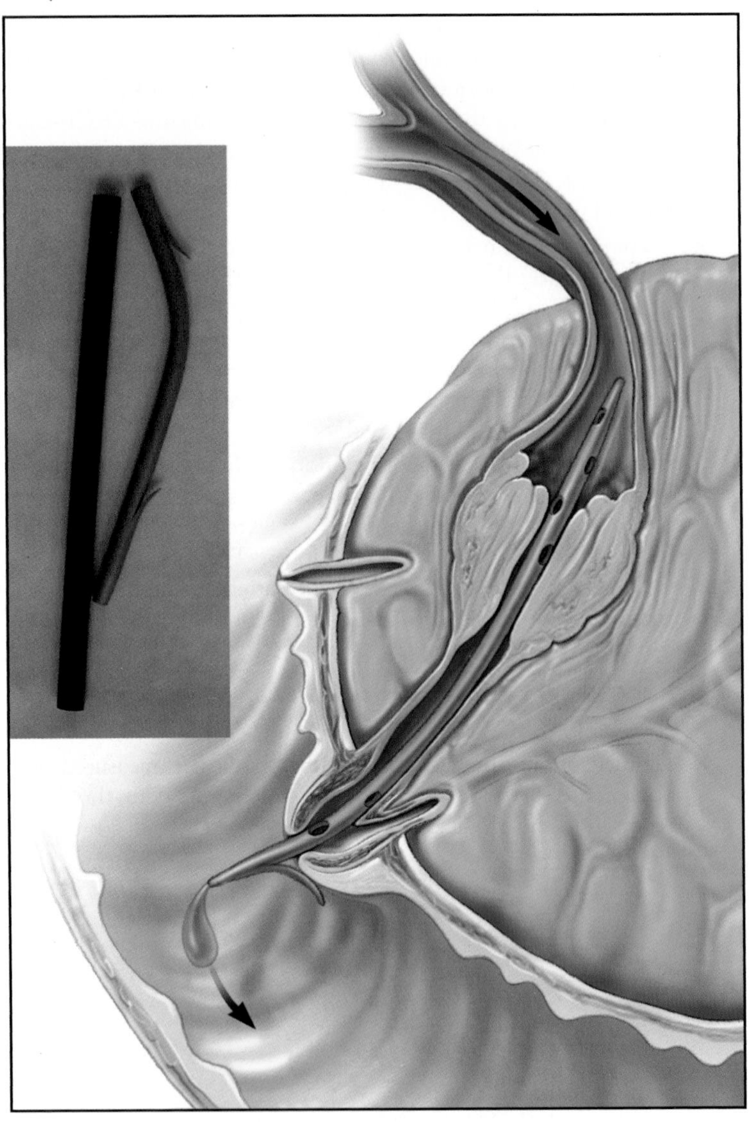

Figure 5-64. Plastic biliary stent across a tumor.

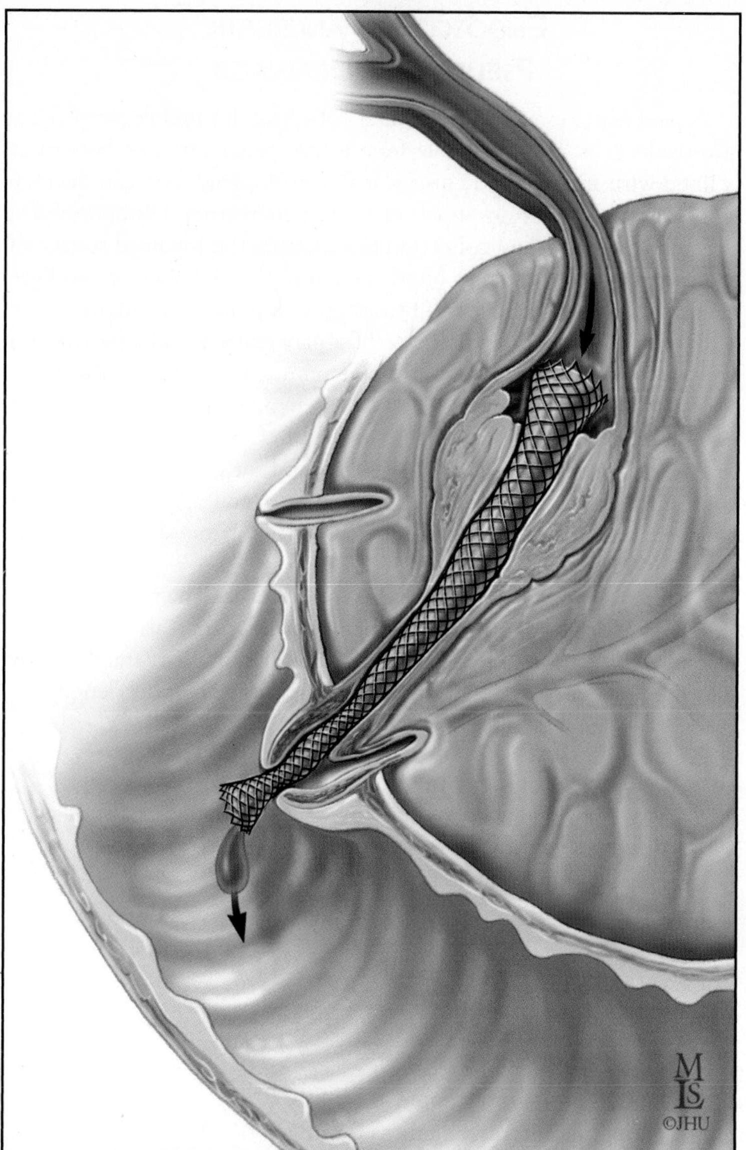

Figure 5-65. Expandable metallic stent across a tumor.

Chapter 5

Endoscopic Pancreatic Pseudocyst Drainage

A pancreatic pseudocyst is a fluid collection located in peripancreatic tissue. It is distinguishable from a true pancreatic cyst because it is lined with inflammatory and scar tissue. A pseudocyst can develop within 6 weeks after an attack of acute pancreatitis. Disruption of a pancreatic duct or fluid collection arising from the inflamed surface of the pancreas may be due to blunt trauma to the abdomen or blockage of the pancreatic duct due to fibrosis, protein plug, or calculous.

Successful endoscopic drainage of a pancreatic pseudocyst requires one of the following criteria: 1) communication between the pseudocyst and main pancreatic duct, as seen on ERCP; 2) endoscopic visualization of a bulge from the pseudocyst. Additionally, it is helpful to have CT imaging, endoscopic ultrasound, or contrast injection to confirm the contact between the pseudocyst and adjacent gastric or duodenal wall prior to attempting transgastric or transduodenal endoscopic drainage.

There are two endoscopic options for drainage. The first is through the pancreatic duct using a pancreatic or nasopancreatic stent. The second is by the insertion of a plastic double pigtail biliary stent directly into the pseudocyst through the wall of the stomach or duodenum.

Equipment

1. Same as for ERCP with sphincterotomy.
2. Side-viewing duodenoscope (may need a therapeutic endoscope if using larger than a 7-Fr stent)
3. Needle-knife sphincterotome (Figure 5-66)

Nursing Implications

Preprocedure

- Same as for ERCP.

Intraprocedure (Figure 5-67)

- Patient positioning: Same as for ERCP.
- Patient monitoring: Same as for ERCP.
- Topical anesthetic: Same as for ERCP.
- Additional comfort measures: Same as for ERCP.

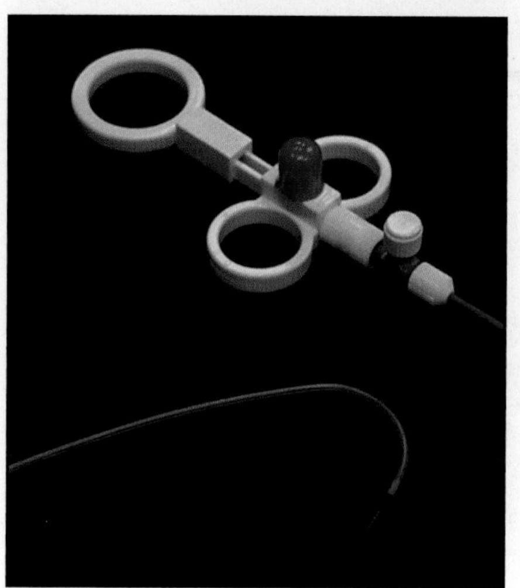

Figure 5-66. Needle-knife sphincterotome.

Postprocedure

- Same as for ERCP.
- Observe for signs of infection (fever, chills, abdominal pain) or hemorrhage (tachycardia, hypotension).

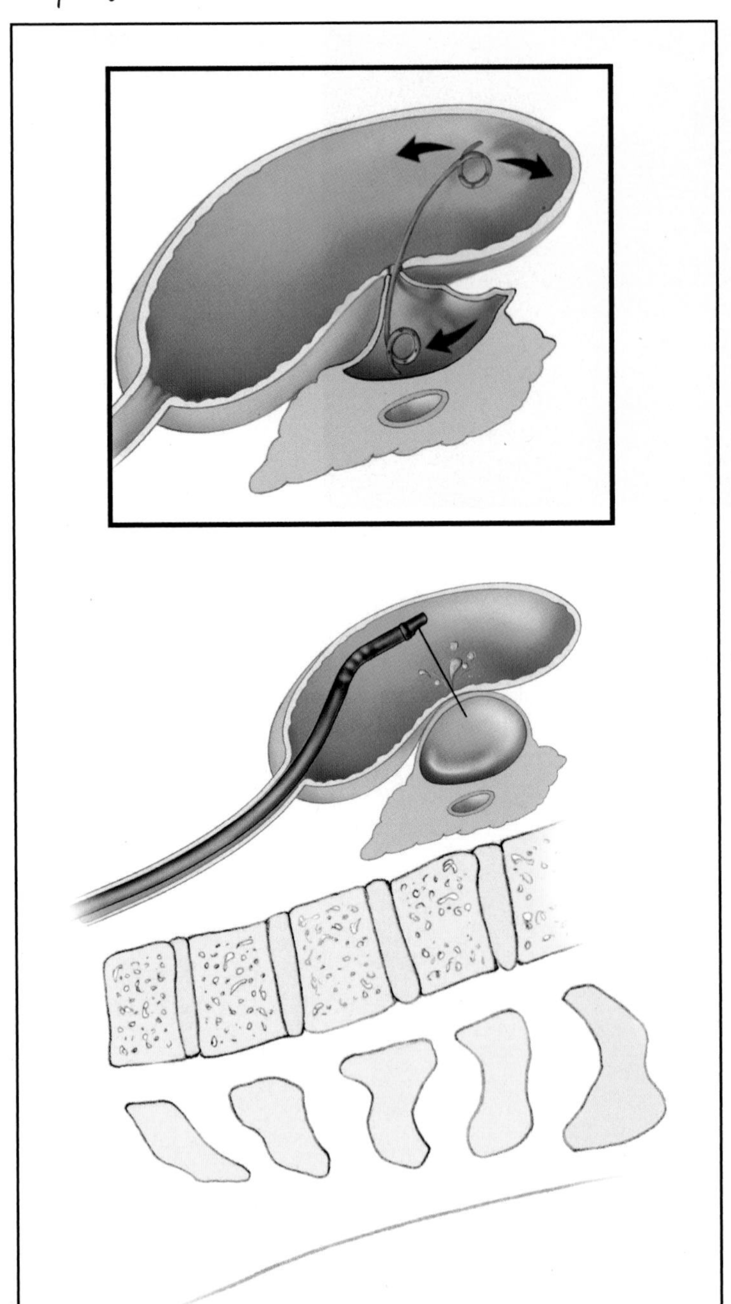

Figure 5-67. Endoscope technique for transgastric pseudocyst drainage.

Biliary Manometry

Biliary manometry refers to the manometric measurement of sphincter of Oddi pressure. This procedure is currently considered the "gold standard" for the diagnosis of sphincter of Oddi dysfunction. Pressure is measured directly with a triple-lumen water-perfused catheter that is passed through the duodenoscope into the bile or pancreatic duct. The proximal end of the catheter is connected to external transducers and a computerized recording device. Sphincter pressures are recorded as the catheter is slowly withdrawn from the duct and stationed within the sphincter zone. The duodenal pressure is taken from the zero reference point when measuring ductal and sphincteric pressures. Abnormalities that may be revealed on manometric studies include elevated basal sphincter pressure, increased frequency of phasic waves, increased proportion of phasic waves propagated in a retrograde direction, and a paradoxical sphincter response to cholecystokinin-octapeptide (CCK-OP).

Equipment

1. Triple-lumen biliary manometry catheter
2. Water perfusion system (pump and transducers)
3. Side-viewing endoscope (duodenoscope) and light source
4. Computer recorder
5. Standard ERCP cannula of physician's choice
6. Water-soluble lubricant
7. Tape (preferably translucent)

Nursing Implications

Preprocedure

- Same as for ERCP.
- The patient must be free of muscle relaxants and opiates for 24 hours prior to the test (these affect sphincter pressure and alter test results).
- Patients on long-term pain medication may be difficult to sedate and may require general anesthesia.
- Duodenal pressures may be monitored with the use of an external cannula (attached to the endoscope using translucent tape applied every 10 cm along the dorsal side).

Intraprocedure

- Patient positioning: Same as for ERCP.
- Patient monitoring: Same as for ERCP.
- Topical anesthetic: Same as for ERCP.
- Additional comfort measures:
  1. Same as for ERCP with sphincterotomy.
  2. Since several pharmacological and hormonal agents influence sphincter of Oddi function, the endoscopist must avoid using glucagon, atropine, morphine, and other opiate analgesics and smooth muscle relaxants.
  3. It is the nurses' responsibility to keep the patient calm and quiet with words of reassurance and light back massage.
- Propofol may be used for deep sedation (Figure 5-68).

Postprocedure

- Same as for ERCP with sphincterotomy.
- Any time manipulation of the bile or pancreatic duct occurs, there is a 1% to 5% risk of causing pancreatitis (symptoms: abdominal pain, vomiting, fever, chills). There is an increased risk for procedure-related pancreatitis (as high as 30%) in sphincter of Oddi manometry, especially if there are prolonged or repeated measurements of the pancreatic duct. The patient should be advised of the potential risks of pancreatitis.
- Nursing measures that may decrease the risk of pancreatitis include:
  1. Conducting periodic cultures of manometry equipment.
  2. Limiting the catheter perfusion rate to 0.25 mL/lumen per minute or less.
  3. Use of aspiration-type manometry catheters when measuring pancreatic sphincter pressure; this type of catheter has two channels for pressure measurements and one channel to aspirate infused fluid and pancreatic juice.

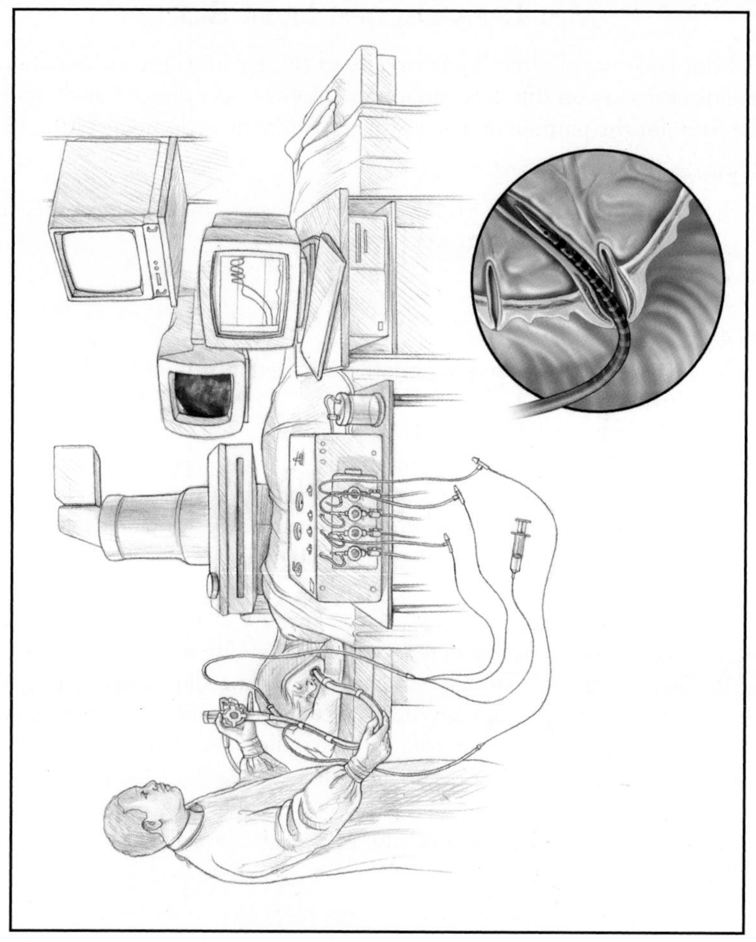

Figure 5-68. Patient set-up for ERCP manometry.

Chapter 5

Mini-Laparoscopic Liver Biopsy

Mini-laparoscopic liver biopsy refers to the laparoscopic examination of lesions or masses on the liver surface and biopsy under direct visualization of the liver, for the purpose of diagnosis and treatment of disorders of the liver.

Equipment

1. Video monitor with photo and video access (includes DVD recorder and printer, mini-lap tower [Figure 5-69])
2. Light source
3. Camera box
4. CO_2 gas tank
5. Laparo Pneu automatic insufflator (Richard Wolf Medical Corp., Vernon Hills, IL)
6. APC unit available if needed
7. Sterile laparoscopic tray: mini fiber laparoscope with outer metal sheath (2 pieces), Veres cannula (metal) (Spectrum Hydro-Med Products, Inc. Los Angeles, CA), laparoscope camera head, flexible light cable, insufflator tubing (disposable), sterile camera drape (used if necessary) (disposable)
8. Prep Tray: (4) sterile drapes, (4) sterile drape clamps (metal), (2) sterile prep solution (ie, Dura prep, Steri prep, or Chlora prep)
9. Biopsy Tray: (2) Tru-cut automated biopsy needles (disposable), 30-cc bottle of 1% lidocaine, sterile bottle of normal saline, 3-cc syringes with #23 needle, #11 scalpel blade with handle, 10-cc leur lock syringes
10. Pack of sterile 4x4 gauze
11. Sterile scissors
12. (2) 3-0 silk and absorbable sutures
13. Hemistat or tweezers

Additional Equipment That May be Needed

1. 2 adhesive dressings or tape
2. Bottles of formalin for biopsy specimens
3. Patient identification label and pathology requisitions
4. Cytology brushes
5. Viral and fungal culture tubes
6. Grounding pad

Nursing Implications

Preprocedure

- Same as for upper endoscopy.
- Reassure patient about various movements in the room and the noises of the equipment.

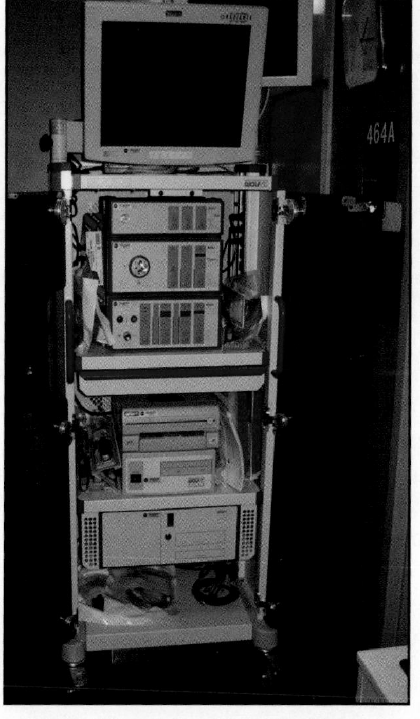

Figure 5-69. Mini-lap tower.

- Prepare the room.
- All equipment listed previously should be carefully inspected and set up for procedure.
  1. The CO_2 gas cylinder should be in the on position, and then turn on the insufflator. The insufflator must be tested to assure maximum level of gas for procedure.
  2. The video system must be tested for proper functioning and patient information entered into the computer.
  3. Sterile gowns, gloves, caps, shoe covers, sterile prep solution, scrub sponges, and sterile towels should be readily available for all staff involved in case needed.
  4. The laparoscopic trays should be opened on a sterile field on a rolling table.
  5. A smaller sterile field should be prepared for the prep trey.
- Patient positioning: Patient should be supine with arms secured to prevent contamination of sterile field.
- Patient monitoring: Follow sedation protocol.

Intraprocedure

- Sedation and monitoring nurse:
  1. Should be at the head of the bed for monitoring the patient and administration of medications.
  2. During insufflation of the peritoneal cavity the monitoring nurse may palpate the chest to check for crepitance, which would indicate passage of gas into the subcutaneous space of the chest. If crepitance is felt, notify physician for reposition of needle.
  3. During insufflation the patient may feel mild discomfort or nausea while the abdominal wall is distending.
  4. Provide medication or comfort measures as needed.
- Circulating assistant:
  1. Should be within easy reach of mini-lap tower and controls for any adjustments during the case.
  2. It is essential that the insufflator monitor be in direct view of the physician at all times to ensure infusions pressures at about 20 to 30 mm/Hg in the peritoneal cavity.
- Scrub nurse to assist MD with the procedure:
  1. She/he should remain sterile through out the case.
  2. As the procedure begins, the scrub nurse will explain to the patient that he/she will feel a sting as the physician anesthetize the skin of the abdomen with lidocaine.
  3. Once the abdomen is distended and laprascope is inserted (by MD) and in place, the scrub nurse will assist physician in attaching the camera head to the laprascope.
  4. After biopsy is obtained the CO_2 is allowed to escape thru the trocar and the abdomen is cleaned of excess blood and sutured by physician if required. Cover with an adhesive bandage.
  5. Assist the physician with taking the biopsy as requested.

Postprocedure

- The patient will be transported to the recovery area for observation for 2 hours or as indicated or ordered by physician.
- Patient should be assessed changes in condition or vital signs.
- Abdominal puncture site should be assessed for leaking of fluid or blood, swelling, or development of hematoma.
- Patient should be assessed for severe abdominal pain, or any complaints of shoulder pain.
- Assess patient for nausea, vomiting, abdominal distention, or fever.
- Notify the physician for any of the above or changes in condition.
- The patient may be discharged home, accompanied by an adult with discharge instructions for liver biopsy (see Appendix 3).

Esophageal Motility Studies

Esophageal motility studies are performed to measure esophageal pressures and contractions. They may be indicated in patients having difficulty swallowing, experiencing noncardiac chest pain, and heartburn. This test measures the pressures within the esophagus by passing a long, thin, flexible manometric catheter (diameter is comparable to a nasogastric tube) into the stomach. The catheter is then pulled back slowly through the lower esophageal sphincter (LES), through the body of the esophagus, and through the upper esophageal sphincter (UES). The transmitters placed every 5 cm on the catheter transmit the pressures to a computer. The computer prints out the information on a tracing in the form of high and low waves.

Equipment

1. Manometry catheter
2. Manometry machine
3. Water-soluble lubricant
4. 8 oz of water with a straw

Nursing Implications

Preprocedure

- The patient should have nothing to eat or drink after midnight prior to the test.
- A medical and surgical history, including medications, should be obtained before the procedure.
- The patient should discontinue use of smooth muscle relaxants or any drugs that would decrease esophageal motility for 72 hours prior to the test.
- The patient's physician should determine whether to discontinue the use of proton pump inhibitors or H2 blockers at least 48 hours before the test (Figure 5-70).

Intraprocedure

- The patient may be sitting on the side of the bed holding a glass of water with a straw for the insertion of the motility catheter.
- The nurse should determine which nostril is more patent by holding each nostril closed and asking the patient to exhale though his or her nose. The more patent nostril should be used.

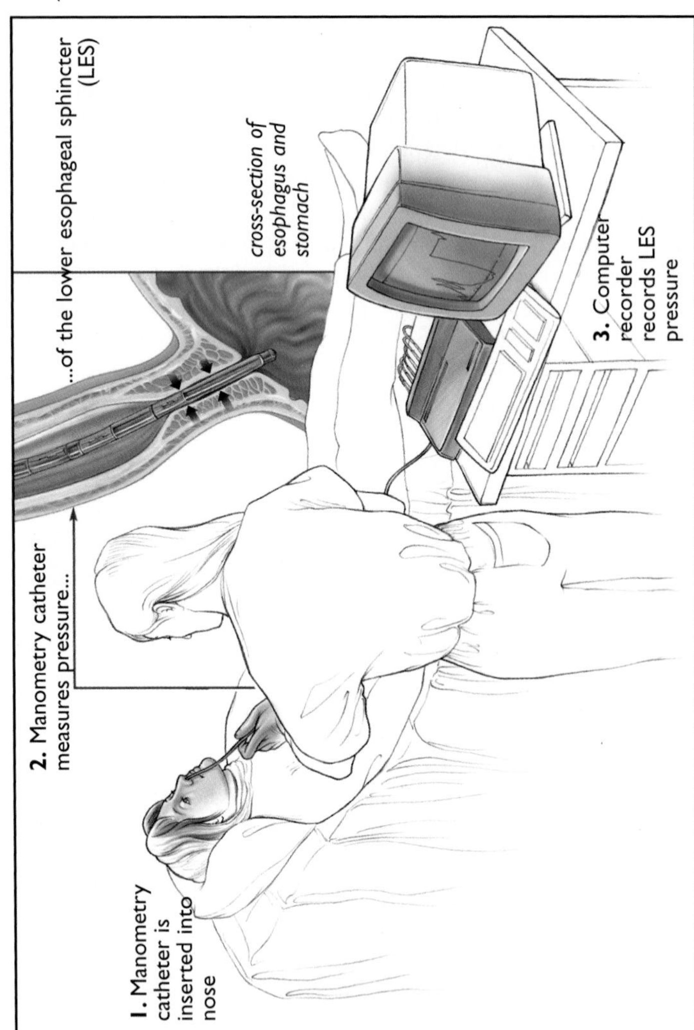

Figure 5-70. Patient set-up for esophageal motility.

- The first 10 cm of the motility catheter should be lubricated with a water-soluble lubricant.
- The nurse should begin inserting the catheter, instructing the patient to start sipping water when he or she feels the tube in the back of his or her throat. The tube can be advanced with each swallow, allowing the peristaltic waves of the esophagus to advance the catheter to the stomach. If insertion is difficult, turning the patient's head to the side changes the position of the esophagus and may facilitate passage of the catheter. Do not try to force the catheter because it may cause esophageal perforation (particularly if the patient has an esophageal diverticulum).
- Once the catheter is in the stomach, the patient is instructed to lie on his or her back with the head and chest elevated (about 30 to 40 degrees).
- The catheter is attached to the computer and slowly withdrawn.
- The patient should remain as still and quiet as possible and avoid swallowing unless instructed to do so. The test takes approximately 45 minutes to complete.

Postprocedure

- Once the tube is removed, the patient may be discharged.
- Normal meals, activities, and medications may be resumed.

Chapter 5

24-Hour pH Monitoring

This test is performed to record the pH (measurement of acidity) in the esophagus over a 24-hour period. Twenty-four-hour pH monitoring is usually performed in conjunction with esophageal motility studies, since the motility tracing is used to determine the placement of the pH probe (5 cm above the LES).

Equipment

1. pH probe and grounding electrode
2. Surgical tape
3. Water-soluble lubricant
4. Digitrapper monitor (MedTronic Inc, Shoreview, Minn) and shoulder strap (computer that collects and assembles reflux data)
5. pH 7 and pH 1 buffer solutions (to calibrate the Digitrapper) (Figure 5-71)

Nursing Implications

Preprocedure

- The patient should have nothing by mouth for at least 8 hours prior to the test.
- The patient's physician should determine whether to discontinue medications that alter pH (eg, H2 blockers, proton pump inhibitors, or other medications).
- A medical/surgical history, including medications, should be obtained prior to the procedure.

Intraprocedure

- The patient may sit on the side of the bed holding a glass of water with a straw for the catheter insertion.
- The first 10 cm of the catheter should be lubricated with a water-soluble lubricant.
- The nurse should determine which nostril is more patent by holding each closed one at a time and asking the patient to exhale through the nose. The more patent nostril should be used.
- The nurse should begin inserting the catheter while instructing the patient to start sipping the water when he or she feels the

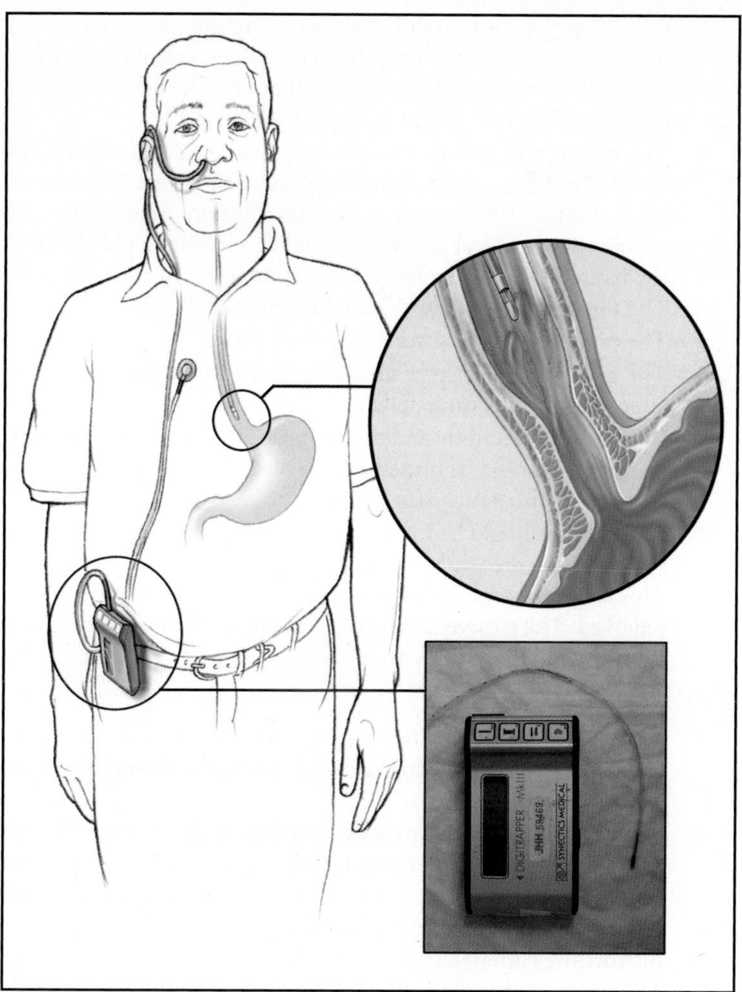

Figure 5-71. Location of ambulatory pH probe in a patient.

tube in the back of his or her throat. The tube can be advanced with each swallow, allowing the peristaltic waves of the esophagus to advance the catheter to the stomach. The position can be confirmed by obtaining an acid pH (below 4).

- ❖ The tube is pulled back into the esophagus to the level of 5 cm above the LES, as determined by the esophageal manometry study. Unless the patient is having constant reflux, the pH should rise to a level above 5. If unable to obtain a pH above 5, the patient should be instructed to drink water to clear the acid. The physician should be notified if this attempt fails.
- ❖ The probe should be securely taped in place.
- ❖ The grounding electrode should be taped to the patient's chest after applying electrode jelly.
- ❖ Connect the electrode and the pH probe to the Digitrapper. The instrument should be turned on and placed in a shoulder strap to be worn by the patient for 24 hours.
- ❖ The patient should be informed that his or her throat might feel scratchy and sore while the tube is in place and after its removal. This is normal and should disappear a few hours after the tube is removed. The patient should have a contact number if the probe is dislodged or questions arise.

Postprocedure

- ❖ The patient should be instructed to keep a diary to record pain and daily mealtime, bedtime, and awake times during the night and in the morning.
- ❖ Normal daily activities may be resumed, with the exception of bathing in a tub or performing strenuous activities. Vigorous exercise could cause the patient to perspire and dislodge the electrode or probe or damage the Digitrapper.
- ❖ Instruct the patient to return after 24 hours to remove the probe. This process takes about 10 to 15 minutes. After probe removal, the patient may resume all normal meals, activities, and medications.

BRAVO pH PROBE PLACEMENT

The Bravo (Medtronic, Minneapolis, MN) probe is also used to diagnose gastroesophageal reflux disease, but is placed during endoscopy. A routine EGD is performed and the physician measures the centimeters from the mouth to 5 cm above the LES. The scope is removed and the Bravo capsule, which is the size of a gel capsule, is inserted into the mouth and down to the point in the esophagus where it will be attached. This is accomplished by a special delivery system. Suction is applied to the esophageal mucosa pulling tissue into the capsule. The physician pushes a button at the proximal end of the delivery system which fires a pin into the suctioned mucosa to hold the capsule against the esophageal wall. The pH is recorded by sending radio telemetry signals to the receiver which is worn on the patient's belt like a pager. After 24 to 48 hours of monitoring, the receiver may be returned via mail or in person and the information is downloaded by an infrared link to a computer. The capsule should pass on its own from the body in several days. The advantages of this system are patient comfort, since there is no uncomfortable tube coming from the patient's nose, and less chance of obtaining false readings, since the patient is more likely to eat and sleep normally.

Equipment

1. Bravo pH receiver
2. Bravo pH capsule (Figure 5-72)
3. Bravo calibration stand
4. Bravo data link
5. 1-AA Lithium/LR6, 1.5 battery
6. Calibration buffer solutions: 7.01 and 1.07
7. Polygram net pH testing application software
8. Sterile water, 1-500cc bottle
9. 70-90% isopropyl alcohol
10. Medela vacuum pump and connecting tubing
11. Same as for EGD

Preprocedure

- Same as for EGD, with the addition of patient being off PPIs for 7 days and Histamine-2 receptor antagonists for at least 2 days.
- Calibrate the Bravo capsule the morning of the procedure according to the manufacturer's instructions.
- Explain diet, activity, and diary instructions to the patient before the procedure because of the sedation used.

Figure 5-72. Bravo capsule.

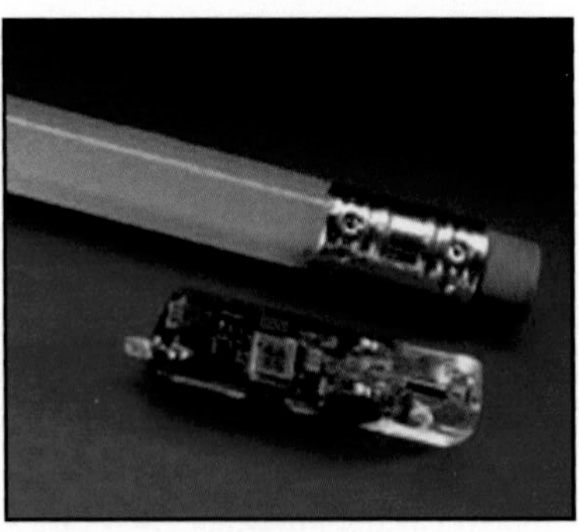

Intraprocedure

- Same as for EGD, with the exception of the special suction set-up used in the Bravo placement. Follow manufacturer's instructions for set-up.

Postprocedure

- Same as for EGD, with the exception of attaching the receiver to the patient's belt before discharge and sending him or her home with written instructions and diary. The diary information is the same as for the pH probe that is not placed endoscopically. The patient needs to be aware that the capsule should pass on it's own a few days, but if the patient develops signs and symptoms of obstruction (eg, abdominal pain or vomiting) he should contact the physician immediately and an abdominal film should be performed.

Capsule Endoscopy

Capsule endoscopy allows the physician to examine the mucosa of the small intestine with the use of a very small video camera, the size of a large vitamin pill, swallowed with a glass of water. The capsule travels through the intestines, via peristaltic waves, capturing pictures at a rate of 14 pictures per second. The images are captured via sensors placed on various points on the patient's abdomen and sent to a data recorder worn on the patient's belt. After 8 hours, the recorder is removed from the patient and then downloaded into a special program on the computer. The physician is able to view all the captured images on the computer and detect the presence of ulcers or bleeding. Capsule endoscopy is used for diagnosing chronic unexplained abdominal pain, diarrhea, bleeding, and anemia of unknown origin. It can also be used to provide information on GI tract motility.

Contraindications of capsule endoscopy are patient's having implantable electrical devices, suspected intestinal obstruction, esophageal swallowing disorders, or strictures.

Equipment

1. Video capsule (Figure 5-73)
2. Data recorder and belt
3. Battery pack
4. Chargers
5. 8 electrodes
6. RAPID (Reporting and processing of images and data) application and software package (Given Imaging Inc., Duluth, GA)
7. Glass of water with a few drops of simethecone

Nursing Implications

Preprocedure

- ❖ Charge the battery pack the evening before the procedure according to the manufacturer's instructions.
- ❖ The morning prior to the procedure, the patient may have a regular breakfast and then clear liquids until 10 pm.
- ❖ Patient should not eat or drink anything after 10 pm the night before the procedure, and should refrain from taking medication for 2 hours before the procedure.
- ❖ Instruct the patient to wear loose fitting clothing.

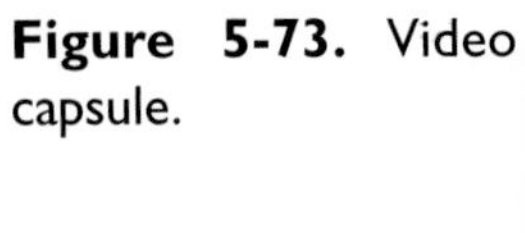

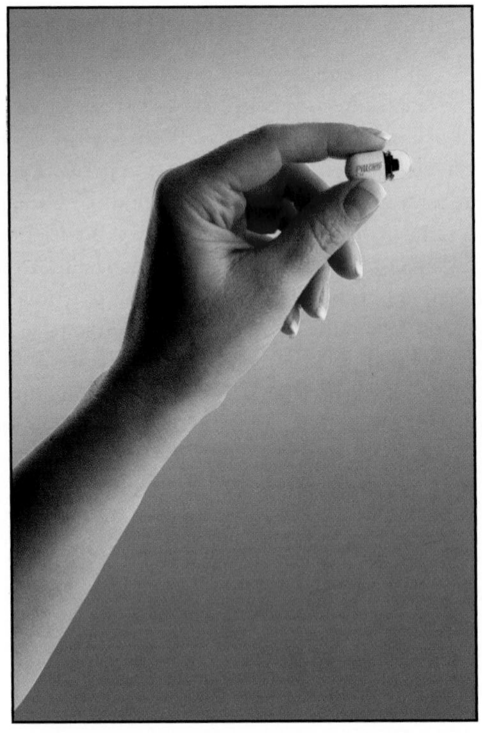

Figure 5-73. Video capsule.

- ❖ If the patient has a hairy abdomen, instruct them to shave an area 6 inches above and 6 inches below the navel in a square.
- ❖ Early the morning of the procedure calibrate the electrodes and download the information into the recorder according to the manufacturer's instructions.
- ❖ Obtain the patient's height, weight, and waist size in inches. Also needed are a brief medical and surgical history, patient allergies, and a review of the contraindications with the patient.
- ❖ Informed consent should be obtained.

Intraprocedure

- ❖ Attach the electrodes and data recorder to the patient as per the manufacturer's instructions.
- ❖ Videotape the patient's name and identifying information; also have patient hold video capsule up to his/her face to take a picture for identification purposes.
- ❖ Have patient swallow the video capsule with a glass of water containing a few drops of simethicone.
- ❖ Patient may leave the area but must return in eight hours or when the video capsule exits the body.

Postprocedure

- ❖ Instruct the patient not to eat or drink anything for 2 hours after the ingestion of the video capsule. A light snack may be ingested after 4 hours. They may resume their regular diet after the test is complete.
- ❖ Inform the patient not to disconnect the belt or suspenders until after the test is finished and to avoid strenuous exercise and bending over while the test is in progress.
- ❖ Have the patient check the blinking light on the recorder every 15 minutes or so to see if the light is still blinking. If it is not, instruct them to return to the unit for further instructions.
- ❖ Patient must check all bowel movements while the test is in progress to see if the capsule has passed prematurely.
- ❖ Patient must return to the unit after 8 hours to have belt and recorder removed.
- ❖ If capsule does not pass within 3 to 4 days, the patient should notify his physician so an abdominal x-ray can be performed.

Chapter 5

Acid Perfusion Test (Bernstein Test)

The acid perfusion or Bernstein test may be used to diagnose gastroesophageal reflux disease (GERD). It is performed in the GI laboratory by alternately infusing normal saline and diluted 0.1 N HCl (hydrochloric acid) into the distal esophagus. The Bernstein test confirms sensitivity to acid in the esophagus.

During the procedure, the patient is blinded to the infusion of 60 to 80 mL of 0.1 N HCl or normal saline. The infusion is introduced into a nasogastric tube (placed at 30 cm) into the esophagus at a rate of 6 to 8 mL/minute. The nurse is responsible for recording the patient's response. Reproduction of the patient's typical symptoms (on two acid infusions) may be interpreted as a positive test response. If this is the case, the physician will most likely treat the patient for GERD.

Equipment

1. Two 1000-mL containers, one containing 1000 cc of normal saline, the other containing 1000 cc of 0.1 N HCl
2. Y-connecting tube that attaches to each bottle and joins to form one that connects to a nasogastric tube
3. 12-Fr nasogastric tube
4. 60-cc catheter-tip syringe
5. Cup of water and a straw
6. Water-soluble lubricant

Nursing Implications

Preprocedure

- The patient should have nothing by mouth after midnight prior to the test.
- The patient must be advised to allow 2 hours for the test (symptoms need to be reproduced at least twice).
- A medical/surgical history should be obtained, documenting medications and allergies.
- The patient's physician should determine whether to discontinue medications that alter pH (eg, H2 blockers, proton pump inhibitors, and other medications). If necessary, medications should be discontinued 2 to 7 days prior to the procedure.

Intraprocedure

- ❖ The patient should be in a sitting position with the bottles of saline and HCl located behind him or her.
- ❖ The patient is asked to swallow sips of water while the lubricated nasogastric tube is inserted through the most patent nostril. If the patient cannot tolerate the nasal tube insertion, it may be inserted through the mouth.
- ❖ Placement of the tube in the stomach is confirmed by using the stethoscope placed on the abdominal area over the stomach to listen for the "swish" of air that is forced through the tube using a 60-cc catheter-tip syringe. The tube is then withdrawn to 30 cm and taped in place.
- ❖ The nasogastric tube is connected to a Y set-up, and the saline drip is initiated. The patient must be watched carefully for symptoms, and reactions should be recorded.
- ❖ The nurse will alternate solutions without the patient's knowledge and record reactions.
- ❖ If symptoms are reproduced with HCl, the nurse should switch back to saline solution until the symptoms subside. Subsequently, symptoms must be reproduced a second time. If symptoms do not subside fully, but only lessen in severity, this must also be accurately recorded.

Postprocedure

- ❖ The tube is removed upon completion of the study and the patient may be discharged.
- ❖ Gargling with warm salt water or using throat lozenges may relieve sore throat symptoms.
- ❖ The patient may resume a normal diet unless otherwise instructed.
- ❖ The physician may prescribe an antacid if the patient's symptoms do not abate.

Chapter 5

Basal Acid Output Test

A basal acid output (BAO) study measures the amount of acid in the stomach after fasting for 8 hours (baseline acid level). This test is performed to evaluate the effectiveness of acid suppression (with proton pump inhibitors, H2 blockers, or surgical vagotomy) and to evaluate the patient for hyperacidity.

Equipment

1. 12-Fr nasogastric tube
2. Intermittent suction set-up
3. 60-cc catheter-tip syringe
4. Stethoscope
5. Water-soluble lubricant
6. Containers for collection of specimens (labeled with date, time, amount)

Nursing Implications

Preprocedure

- ❖ The patient should have nothing by mouth after midnight prior to the test.
- ❖ A medical/surgical history, including medications, should be obtained prior to the procedure.
- ❖ The patient's physician should determine whether to discontinue medications that alter pH (eg, H2 blockers, proton pump inhibitors, or other medications). If necessary, medications should be discontinued 2 to 7 days prior to the procedure.
- ❖ If the test is being done to evaluate the effectiveness of treatment, medications should be taken as prescribed until the morning of the test.

Intraprocedure

- ❖ The patient should sit on the side of the bed for insertion of the nasogastric tube.
- ❖ The first 10 cm of the tube should be lubricated. No water should be sipped, as it may alter the study results.
- ❖ Swallowing facilitates insertion of the tube.
- ❖ Placement of the tube in the stomach is confirmed by using a stethoscope to listen for the "swish" of air that is forced through the tube using a 60-cc catheter-tip syringe.

- ❖ Once placement is confirmed, stomach contents should be suctioned and placed in a labeled container (baseline specimen). Subsequent specimens should be collected at 15-minute intervals for a total of four times during the study and labeled appropriately.
- ❖ The tube should be removed after the last specimen has been obtained, and the patient may be discharged.
- ❖ Specimens should be sent to the lab for analysis. Specimens are evaluated for amount, color, consistency, pH, hydrogen ion concentration, and total acid content. This information is forwarded to the physician.

Postprocedure

- ❖ The patient may be discharged and may resume regular diet, medications, and activities.

Chapter 5

Secretin Stimulation Study

The secretin stimulation study is performed in the GI laboratory to detect the presence of Zollinger-Ellison syndrome (gastrinoma). This is a nonbeta islet cell tumor of the pancreas, which causes large amounts of gastrin to be secreted into the blood stream. Three primary characteristics of this disease are severe peptic ulcer formation in unusual locations, gastric hypersecretion of gigantic proportions, and nonspecific islet cell tumors of the pancreas. Thickened folds of the stomach and chronic diarrhea are also prominent symptoms, but may be indicative of other diseases. Most patients with gastrinoma present with complaints of abdominal pain. During the secretin stimulation test, a baseline blood level is drawn. Then, secretin 2 cu/kg is injected intravenously. Blood samples are drawn at intervals of 2, 5, 10, 15, and 30 minutes. In patients with gastrinoma, peak serum levels occur at 2 to 5 minutes and are normal again at 15 minutes.

Equipment

1. 20-g angiocatheter or larger and heparin lock
2. Six red-topped tubes for blood collection
3. Tourniquet
4. Container filled with ice (10-oz styrofoam cup)
5. Vials of secretin (enough for 2 cu/kg of body weight)
6. Vials of injectable saline to reconstitute secretin
7. Seven 10-cc syringes (if a Vacutainer [Becton, Dickinson & Co, Franklin Lakes, NJ] is used, only one 10-cc syringe is required)
8. Watch or timer
9. Alcohol wipes and 2x2 gauze pads with tape

Nursing Implications

Preprocedure

- Prior to scheduling, a baseline gastrin level should be obtained.
- The patient should have nothing by mouth after midnight prior to the test.
- Discontinue proton pump inhibitors and H2 blockers 72 hours prior to testing.
- Obtain a brief medical history along with allergies and medications.

Intraprocedure

- The patient may sit in a chair or lie supine depending upon his or her preference.
- An intravenous line is placed with a 20-g angiocatheter or larger and a heparin lock placed onto the angiocatheter. This facilitates access for blood drawing. There is no need to use heparin in between the blood draws, flushing with saline is sufficient to keep the line patent.
- Apply the tourniquet for each blood draw and remove it in between blood draws.
- Draw a baseline blood level, and then inject secretin 2 cu/kg slowly over 1 to 2 minutes.
- If the patient has any untoward reaction to the secretin, stop the test and call the physician immediately. Reactions to secretin are very rare, but it has been reported that a rash or hives may occur at the injection site.
- Blood samples should be drawn at intervals of 2, 5, 10, 15, and 30 minutes.
- All vials of collected blood should be kept on ice until delivery to the appropriate laboratory for analysis.

Postprocedure

- After the test is complete, the intravenous line should be removed and the patient may be discharged.
- The patient should be instructed to call his or her physician if the injection site becomes red or swollen.

BIBLIOGRAPHY

Bayless TM, ed. *Current Therapy in Gastroenterology and Liver Disease*. 3rd ed. Philadelphia, Pa: BC Decker; 1990.

Gastrointestinal Endoscopy Online. 1998;48(6). Available at: http://www.harcourthealth.com/scripts/om.dll/serve?action=searchDB&searchDBfor=iss&id=jge980486&target=. Accessed April 2002.

Johns Hopkins Hospital. *Johns Hopkins Policy and Procedure Manual for GI Endoscopy*. Baltimore, Md: Author; 2000.

Johns Hopkins Hospital. *Johns Hopkins Conscious Sedation Protocol*. Baltimore, Md: Author; 2000.

Johns Hopkins Hospital. *Johns Hopkins Interdisciplinary Clinical Practice Manual*. Baltimore, Md: Author; 1998.

Johns Hopkins Drug Information Service. Personal communication. July 2001.

Kiesslich, R, et al. Confocal laser endomicroscopy. *Gastrointestinal Endosocopy Clinics of North America*. 2005;15:715-731.

McNally PR, ed. *GI/Liver Secrets*. Philadelphia, Pa: Hanley & Belfus Inc; 1996.

Physicians Desk Reference. 54th ed. Montvale, NJ: Medical Economics Co; 2000.

Salmore R. Our heritage: a history of gastroenterology and gastroenterology nursing. *Gastroenterology Nursing*. 1998;21:2;40-43.

Bibliography

Schindler G. Assisting at gastroscopy. *Bulletin of Gastrointestinal Endoscopy*. 1964;11:10-12.

Society of Gastroenterology Nurses and Associates Inc. *Buyer's Guide and Pharmaceutical Reference*. 7th ed. Philadelphia, Pa: Lippincott, Williams & Wilkins; 2001:45-56.

Society of Gastroenterology Nurses and Associates Inc. SGNA guidelines for nursing care of the patient receiving sedation and analgesia in the gastrointestinal endoscopy setting. *Gastroenterology Nursing*. 2000;23(3):125-138.

Society of Gastroenterology Nurses and Associates Inc. Standards of infection control in reprocessing of flexible gastrointestinal endoscopes. *Gastroenterology Nursing*. 2000;23(4):172-179.

Society of Gastroenterology Nurses and Associates Inc. Position statement, role delineation of the registered nurse in a staff position in gastroenterology and/or endoscopy. *Gastroenterology Nursing*. 1998;21(2):99-100.

Tsujikawa, Y, et al. Novel single-balloon enteroscopy for diagnosis and treatment of the small intestine: preliminary experiences. *Endoscopy*. 2007;12:18058613.

Yaster M, Krane EJ, Kaplan RF, Cote CJ, Lappe DG. *Pediatric Pain Management and Sedation Handbook*. St. Louis, Mo: Mosby; 1997.

Appendix 1

Patient Preparation for Endoscopic Procedures

Upper Endoscopic Procedures

- The patient should have nothing by mouth for at least 8 hours prior to the procedure.
- If the procedure entails dilation, cutting, biopsy of tissue, or the patient has a known coagulopathy, coagulation studies should be available and the patient should be advised, on the discretion of the physician, to refrain from taking aspirin, ibuprofen, or anticoagulants for 1 week prior to the procedure.
- If ERCP with sphincterotomy or PEG placement is performed, the patient should receive prophylactic antibiotics 1 hour prior to the procedure.
- Antibiotic prophylaxis is dependent upon the procedure to be performed and the discretion of the physician: for patients with prosthetic valves, history of endocarditis, pulmonary shunts, synthetic vascular grafts, mitral valve prolapse with insufficiency, cardiomyopathy, congenital cardiac anomalies, cirrhosis and ascites, and those who are immunocompromised (see Antibiotic Prophylaxis Chart in Chapter 4).

Lower Endoscopic Procedures

- Bowel preparation may be accomplished by using several different methods or a combination of methods:

1. Lavage method: an electrolyte lavage solution (4 L) is given at the rate of 1 to 2 L per hour after a short period of dietary restriction (light nonfibrous lunch and clear liquid supper). If the patient cannot tolerate large amounts of oral fluid, a nasogastric tube may be inserted and the fluid poured through it. No carbohydrate-containing food or fluid should be ingested prior to or with the lavage fluid to prevent excessive sodium absorption. The solutions will not add to the circulating blood volume if used correctly and should be safe in those patients with congestive heart failure, renal impairment, or who might be subject to enhanced absorption of phosphate or sodium.
2. Enema method: Enema until clear in combination with clear liquids or other residue-free diets for 24 to 48 hours. The enemas may be preceded by an oral cathartic such as Citrate of Magnesia. The drawbacks to this method are that it demands considerable time and can cause dehydration and/or hypovolemia if not balanced by adequate oral or intravenous intake, especially in the elderly or in those with cardiopulmonary or renal disease. In debilitated patients or those with partially obstructing colonic lesions, inflammatory bowel disease, or massive lower GI bleed, this method may be impractical and dangerous.
3. Fleet enemas in combination with Citrate of Magnesia are used for flexible sigmoidoscopy. If the patient has been on clear liquids, Fleet enemas alone may be sufficient.
4. Oral saline cathartics (Fleet phosphosoda; Johnson & Johnson Merck, Fort Washington, PA) in combination with suppositories (Dulcolax; Boehringer Ingelheim, Canada) and/or Fleet enemas may be used as an alternative to oral lavage and tap water enemas. This method may be more palatable than the oral lavage method because it requires ingestion of much less fluid. Your health care professional should be made aware if you are on a low salt diet, use diuretics for high blood pressure or arthritis, have heart problems or seizures, have a history of kidney problems, or are pregnant or nursing.

❖ The patient should have nothing by mouth except water until just before the procedure unless general anesthesia is being used, in which case he or she should have nothing by mouth 8 hours prior to the procedure.

Appendix 2

Complications of Endoscopic Procedures

Although complications during endoscopic procedures are uncommon, it is important to maintain adequate documentation and strict adherence to the policies and procedures of the unit and hospital in order to provide optimal patient safety.

Preprocedure

- ❖ All patients should be aware of the risks of the procedure being performed.
- ❖ This is accomplished in writing with an informed consent. The physician explains the reasons for the procedure as well as the risks and possible complications prior to sedation. Any questions the patient may have should be addressed at this time.
- ❖ If the patient is not willing to accept the risks of the procedure, he or she has the right to decline having the procedure performed. The physician is compelled to communicate the risks of not having the procedure and alternative treatments that may be available to the patient.
- ❖ The nurse's responsibility in informed consent is to witness the patient's signature and to answer any other questions the patient may have concerning the procedure.
- ❖ The nurse may act as the patient advocate in relaying any patient fears or concerns to the physician so that he or she may allay them.

INTRAPROCEDURE

- ❖ Complications that may occur during upper endoscopic procedures are:
  1. Perforation that may require surgery
  2. Bleeding
  3. Aspiration pneumonia
  4. In rare cases the lidocaine spray used for topical anesthesia of the throat may cause methemoglobinemia, which is an altered state of hemoglobin in which the ferrous irons of the heme are oxidized to the ferric state. The ferric hemes of methemoglobin are unable to bind oxygen. As a result the oxygen delivery to the tissues is impaired. Therefore, when spraying the patient's throat care should be taken to use the least amount of lidocaine necessary for numbing the throat.
  5. Untoward reaction to sedation or other medication given during the procedure
  6. Shock
  7. Death
- ❖ The nurse's role, should a complication occur, is one of quick recognition of signs and symptoms and communication to the physician. He or she must anticipate the proper sequence of orders the physician will give and act quickly to execute the orders.
- ❖ Standard resuscitation measures should be instituted if there is hemodynamic instability.
- ❖ Perforation during the procedure is usually recognizable by both the physician and the nurse by visualization of unfamiliar structures during the procedure.
- ❖ When perforation is observed, the physician will direct the nurse to do the following:
  1. Immediately abort the procedure.
  2. Monitor vital signs closely.
  3. Obtain blood from the patient for blood type and cross-match for the possibility of transfusion; the physician may order other blood tests to be taken at this time (ie, complete blood count with differential and liver chemistries).
  4. If the patient is conscious, explain what has happened and keep him or her calm and informed.
  5. Obtain x-rays of the affected area.

6. Start intravenous antibiotics.
7. Obtain a surgical consult and start the admission process.
8. Proceed with pain management as needed.
9. Accurately document all events, including date and time, and without bias or finger pointing.
10. Keep the patient's family informed of events that are taking place.

❖ When aspiration is suspected, the physician may direct the nurse to:
1. Obtain a chest x-ray.
2. Start intravenous antibiotics.
3. Monitor vital signs closely, especially oxygen saturation; nasal cannula oxygen should remain at 2 L and should be adjusted as necessary.
4. If the patient is conscious, allay fears and explain what is being done.
5. Start the admission process.
6. Accurately document all events, including date and time, and without bias or finger pointing.
7. Keep the patient's family informed of events that are taking place.

❖ When bleeding is visualized on the screen, the nurse should:
1. Prepare the bipolar cautery (BICAP) for use and prepare epinephrine for injection.
2. If bleeding is not controlled, start a normal saline or lactated Ringers solution and run at 200 cc/hour.
3. Obtain blood from the patient for type and cross-match for the possibility of transfusion; the physician may order other blood tests at this time (ie, complete blood count, serum electrolytes).
4. Obtain a surgical consult.
5. Monitor vital signs closely.
6. If the patient is conscious, explain what has happened and keep the patient calm and informed.
7. Start the admission process.
8. Accurately document all events, including date and time, and without bias or finger pointing.
9. Keep the patient's family informed of the events that are taking place.

- When an adverse medication reaction occurs, the nurse should:
  1. Prepare the reversal medication if necessary and administer on the order of the physician.
  2. Monitor the patient closely for respiratory or cardiac arrest.
  3. Have all emergency equipment readily available.
  4. If the patient is conscious, explain what has happened and keep him or her calm and informed.
  5. Accurately document all events, including date and time, and without bias or finger pointing.
  6. Keep the patient's family informed of events that are taking place.
- Complications for lower endoscopic procedures are the same as for upper endoscopic procedures.
  1. Vasovagal reactions may occur following a colonoscopy or combination of colonoscopy and EGD. The symptoms of this reaction are:
     - Low blood pressure
     - Tachycardia
     - Dizziness
     - May produce loss of consciousness and shock
  2. At the sign of vasovagal reaction, the nurse should:
     - Increase rate of the intravenous normal saline solution
     - Place patient flat or in the Trendelenburg position
     - Notify physician immediately
     - Monitor patient's vital signs closely every 5 minutes until they stabilize
     - Usually vasovagal reactions are transient, but if it becomes more severe the patient may need to be hospitalized
     - Accurately document all events, including date and time, and without bias or finger pointing

POSTPROCEDURE

- Not all complications present themselves during the procedure. The patient may begin to exhibit signs of perforation, aspiration, bleeding, cardiopulmonary distress, and vasovagal reactions in the recovery phase. If this occurs, the same procedures are followed as if it happened during the procedure. The physician should be notified immediately if the nurse observes any abnormal changes in the patient's condition.

- After ERCP, pancreatitis may occur:
  1. If the patient exhibits signs of severe abdominal pain, fever, chills, or vomiting, the physician should be notified immediately.
  2. Antibiotics may be ordered.
  3. Intravenous fluid as per physician's orders.
  4. The patient should not have anything to eat or drink.
  5. The admission process should be started.
  6. Monitor the patient closely.
  7. Keep family members informed of the treatment plan.
  8. Accurately document all events, including date and time, without bias or finger pointing.
  9. Explain what is happening to the patient to allay his or her fears.
- Complications for PEG placement are the same as for upper endoscopy with the exception of infection:
  1. If foul-smelling, purulent drainage is observed around the G-tube site, the physician should be notified.
  2. Document the condition of the G-tube site with time and date.
  3. Document pain level and medicate as necessary.
  4. Intravenous or oral antibiotics may be ordered.
  5. The physician may choose to remove and replace the tube.

Appendix 3

DISCHARGE INSTRUCTIONS FOR ENDOSCOPIC PROCEDURES

Esophagogastroduodenoscopy (EGD) discharge instructions should include:

- ❖ Type of procedure and date performed.
- ❖ Name and phone number of the physician who performed the procedure.
- ❖ Contact phone number in case of emergency.
- ❖ Instructions for follow-up appointments or phone calls.
- ❖ If the patient develops severe epigastric pain, vomits blood, has a temperature of 101°F or higher, or becomes lightheaded or dizzy, the physician should be notified or the patient should be instructed to go to the nearest emergency room.
- ❖ No alcohol or tranquilizers should be consumed for 24 hours unless the physician states otherwise.
- ❖ Light diet progressing to regular diet should be followed by the patient as tolerated unless the physician specifies differently.
- ❖ If the patient has a sore throat after the procedure, he or she may be instructed to use throat lozenges or gargle with warm salt water for relief.
- ❖ If the intravenous site becomes painful, red, or swollen, the patient should contact his or her physician.
- ❖ No driving or strenuous activity should take place for 24 hours. The patient should be in the company of another person for at least 24 hours.
- ❖ The patient should be advised to avoid the use of aspirin or NSAIDs for several days after polyp removal, as directed by the physician.

- The instructions should be completed in duplicate and signed and dated by the patient or responsible party and the nurse.

Colonoscopy discharge instructions should include:

- Type of procedure and date performed.
- Name and phone number of the physician who performed the procedure.
- Contact phone number in case of emergency.
- Instructions for follow-up appointments or phone calls.
- If the patient develops severe lower abdominal pain, distention, or rectal bleeding (a toilet bowl full of blood and clots), develops a temperature of 101°F or higher, or becomes lightheaded or dizzy, the physician should be notified or the patient should be instructed to go to the nearest emergency room.
- No alcohol or tranquilizers should be consumed for 24 hours unless the physician states otherwise.
- Light progressing to regular diet should be followed as tolerated by the patient unless a polyp is removed, in which case a low-fiber diet is suggested for 24 hours to prevent mechanical abrasion to the polypectomy site.
- The patient may expect to be distended and bloated for the remainder of the day due to the insufflation of air into the bowel.
- Contact the physician if the intravenous site becomes red, swollen, or painful.
- No driving or strenuous activity should take place for 24 hours. The patient should be in the company of another person for at least 24 hours.
- The patient should be advised to avoid the use of aspirin or NSAIDs for several days after polyp removal, as directed by the physician.
- The instructions should be completed in duplicate and signed and dated by the patient or responsible party and the nurse.

Sigmoidoscopy discharge instructions should include:

- Type of procedure and date performed.
- Name and phone number of the physician who performed the procedure.
- Contact phone number in case of emergency.

- ❖ Instructions for follow-up appointments or phone calls.
- ❖ If the patient develops severe lower abdominal pain, distention, or rectal bleeding (a toilet bowl full of blood and clots), develops a temperature of 101°F or higher, or becomes lightheaded or dizzy, the physician must be notified or the patient should be instructed to go to the nearest emergency room.
- ❖ No alcohol, tranquilizers, or driving for 24 hours unless the physician states otherwise (only if sedation is used).
- ❖ The patient may expect to be distended and bloated for the rest of the day due to the insufflation of air into the bowel.
- ❖ The patient should be advised to avoid the use of aspirin or NSAIDs for several days after polyp removal, as directed by the physician.
- ❖ The instructions should be completed in duplicate and signed and dated by the patient or responsible party and the nurse.

ERCP discharge instructions should include:

- ❖ Type of procedure and date performed.
- ❖ Name and phone number of the physician who performed the procedure.
- ❖ Contact phone number in case of emergency.
- ❖ Instructions for follow-up appointments or phone calls.
- ❖ If the patient develops severe epigastric pain and vomiting, vomits blood, has a temperature of 101°F or higher, becomes lightheaded or dizzy, or becomes jaundiced, the physician should be notified or the patient should be instructed to go to the nearest emergency room.
- ❖ No alcohol or tranquilizers should be consumed for 24 hours unless the physician states otherwise.
- ❖ Light diet progressing to regular diet should be followed as tolerated by the patient unless the physician specifies otherwise. If a sphincterotomy is performed, the patient should have nothing by mouth with the exception of ice chips for the remainder of the day, progressing to a liquid diet as tolerated.
- ❖ If the patient has a sore throat after the procedure, he or she may be instructed to use throat lozenges or gargle with warm salt water for relief.
- ❖ If the intravenous site becomes painful, red, or swollen, the patient should contact his or her physician.

- No driving or strenuous activity for 24 hours. The patient should be in the company of another person for at least 24 hours.
- The patient should be advised to avoid the use of aspirin or NSAIDs for several days after polyp removal, as directed by the physician.
- The instructions should be completed in duplicate and signed and dated by the patient or responsible party and the nurse.

Mini-Lap discharge instructions should include:

- Type of procedure and date performed.
- Name and phone number of the physician who performed the procedure.
- Contact phone number in case of emergency.
- Instructions for follow-up appointments or phone calls.
- Patient should not drive, operate heavy machinery, or sign legal documents after the administration of moderate sedation for at least 24 hours and should be in the company of another person for 24 hours.
- Patient should be instructed to not lift anything heavy for 48 hours.
- Diet may be as tolerated, avoiding foods that normally cause the patient to have more gas.
- No tub baths for one week, showers are allowed.
- No blood thinners, NSAIDS, or aspirin for 24 hours.
- Contact the physician if any of the following occur:
  1. Redness, soreness or purulent drainage from IV site
  2. An increase in abdominal pain and/or girth
  3. Weakness, dizziness, or lightheadedness
  4. Increase of bloody drainage from puncture site
  5. Nausea, vomiting, or fever

OSHA Guidelines for Cleaning Room Air Quality

- Cleaning rooms in which glutaraldehyde is to be used must be well ventilated and large enough to ensure adequate dilution of vapor, with a minimum air exchange rate of 10 air changes per hour.
- All employees who may be exposed to above the ceiling threshold limit value (TLV) of 0.05 ppm should use appropriate respirators for glutaraldehyde vapor during routine or emergency work.
- Ideally, install local exhaust ventilation, such as properly functioning laboratory fume hoods (capture velocity of at least 100 feet per minute), to control vapor.
- Keep glutaraldehyde baths under a fume hood where possible.
- Use only enough glutaraldehyde to perform the required disinfecting procedure.
- Store glutaraldehyde in closed containers in well-ventilated areas. Air-tight containers are available. Post signs to remind staff to replace lids after using product.
- Use specially designed, mobile, compact, disinfectant soaking stations to facilitate sterilization of heat sensitive equipment such as endoscopes or GI scopes. These soaking stations provide an enclosed area for sterilizing trays and remove fumes from glutaraldehyde and other disinfectants.

Appendix 5

Equipment Manufacturers

The following is a brief list of manufacturers of endoscopic equipment and accessories. A complete list may be found in the Society of Gastroenterology Nurses and Associate's *Buyer's Guide and Pharmaceutical Reference*.

Boston Scientific Corporation
Microvasive Endoscopy
Phone: (800) 225-3226
Website: www.bostonscientific.com

Fujinon Inc
Phone: (800) 385-4666, ext 320
Website: www.fujinon.com

Medovations
Phone: (800) 558-6408
Website: www.medovations.com
Email: medo@medovations.com

MedTronics Functional Diagnostics
Phone: (800) 227-3191
Website: www.medtronic.com
Email: john.gifford@medtronic.com

Appendix 5

Olympus America Inc
Phone: (800) 645-8160
Website: www.olympus.com

Pentax Precision Instrument Corp
Phone: (800) 431-5880
Website: www.pentaxmedical.com

US Endoscopy Group
Phone: (800) 769-8226
Website: www.usendoscopy.com
Email: info@usendoscopy.com

Welch Allyn Protocol
Phone: (800) 289-2500
Website: www.welchallyn.com

Wilson Cook Medical Inc
Phone: (800) 245-4717
Website: www.cookgroup.com

Appendix 6

Web Resources

American Society for Gastrointestinal Endoscopy
www.asge.org

Bard Medical Division
www.bardmedical.com

The DAVE Project
http://daveproject.org

Diprivan Injectable Emulsion
www.diprivan.com

ERBE
www.erbe-med.com

Ethicon Endo-Surgery, Inc.
www.inscope.com

Fleet Phosphosoda
www.phosphosoda.com

Given Imaging
http://givenimaging.com

Hemorrhoid Relief Center
http://www.seekrelief.com

Johns Hopkins Gastroenterology and Hepatology Resource Center
www.hopkins-gi.org

Medtronic
www.medtronic.com

MUSC Pharmacy Services
http://www.musc.edu/pharmacy-services/medusepol/SEDATION.pdf

National Institutes of Diabetes, Digestive, and Kidney Diseases
www.niddk.nih.gov/health/health.htm

National Library of Medicine Pub Med
www.ncbi.nlm.nih.gov/PubMed/

NDO Surgical
www.ndosurgical.com

OSHA
www.osha.gov

RXmed
www.rxmed.com

The Society of Gastroenterology Nurses and Associates
www.sgna.org

UpToDate
www.uptodate.com

Wikipedia
http://en.wikipedia.org

INDEX

Index

Index